ANTICHOLINERGIC AGENTS IN THE UPPER AND LOWER AIRWAYS

LUNG BIOLOGY IN HEALTH AND DISEASE

Executive Editor

Claude Lenfant
*Director, National Heart, Lung and Blood Institute
National Institutes of Health
Bethesda, Maryland*

1. Immunologic and Infectious Reactions in the Lung, *edited by Charles H. Kirkpatrick and Herbert Y. Reynolds*
2. The Biochemical Basis of Pulmonary Function, *edited by Ronald G. Crystal*
3. Bioengineering Aspects of the Lung, *edited by John B. West*
4. Metabolic Functions of the Lung, *edited by Y. S. Bakhle and John R. Vane*
5. Respiratory Defense Mechanisms (in two parts), *edited by Joseph D. Brain, Donald F. Proctor, and Lynne M. Reid*
6. Development of the Lung, *edited by W. Alan Hodson*
7. Lung Water and Solute Exchange, *edited by Norman C. Staub*
8. Extrapulmonary Manifestations of Respiratory Disease, *edited by Eugene Debs Robin*
9. Chronic Obstructive Pulmonary Disease, *edited by Thomas L. Petty*
10. Pathogenesis and Therapy of Lung Cancer, *edited by Curtis C. Harris*
11. Genetic Determinants of Pulmonary Disease, *edited by Stephen D. Litwin*
12. The Lung in the Transition Between Health and Disease, *edited by Peter T. Macklem and Solbert Permutt*
13. Evolution of Respiratory Processes: A Comparative Approach, *edited by Stephen C. Wood and Claude Lenfant*
14. Pulmonary Vascular Diseases, *edited by Kenneth M. Moser*
15. Physiology and Pharmacology of the Airways, *edited by Jay A. Nadel*
16. Diagnostic Techniques in Pulmonary Disease (in two parts), *edited by Marvin A. Sackner*
17. Regulation of Breathing (in two parts), *edited by Thomas F. Hornbein*
18. Occupational Lung Diseases: Research Approaches and Methods, *edited by Hans Weill and Margaret Turner-Warwick*
19. Immunopharmacology of the Lung, *edited by Harold H. Newball*
20. Sarcoidosis and Other Granulomatous Diseases of the Lung, *edited by Barry L. Fanburg*
21. Sleep and Breathing, *edited by Nicholas A. Saunders and Colin E. Sullivan*

22. *Pneumocystis carinii* Pneumonia: Pathogenesis, Diagnosis, and Treatment, *edited by Lowell S. Young*
23. Pulmonary Nuclear Medicine: Techniques in Diagnosis of Lung Disease, *edited by Harold L. Atkins*
24. Acute Respiratory Failure, *edited by Warren M. Zapol and Konrad J. Falke*
25. Gas Mixing and Distribution in the Lung, *edited by Ludwig A. Engel and Manuel Paiva*
26. High-Frequency Ventilation in Intensive Care and During Surgery, *edited by Graziano Carlon and William S. Howland*
27. Pulmonary Development: Transition from Intrauterine to Extrauterine Life, *edited by George H. Nelson*
28. Chronic Obstructive Pulmonary Disease: Second Edition, Revised and Expanded, *edited by Thomas L. Petty*
29. The Thorax (in two parts), *edited by Charis Roussos and Peter T. Macklem*
30. The Pleura in Health and Disease, *edited by Jacques Chrétien, Jean Bignon, and Albert Hirsch*
31. Drug Therapy for Asthma: Research and Clinical Practice, *edited by John W. Jenne and Shirley Murphy*
32. Pulmonary Endothelium in Health and Disease, *edited by Una S. Ryan*
33. The Airways: Neural Control in Health and Disease, *edited by Michael A. Kaliner and Peter J. Barnes*
34. Pathophysiology and Treatment of Inhalation Injuries, *edited by Jacob Loke*
35. Respiratory Function of the Upper Airway, *edited by Oommen P. Mathew and Giuseppe Sant'Ambrogio*
36. Chronic Obstructive Pulmonary Disease: A Behavioral Perspective, *edited by A. John McSweeny and Igor Grant*
37. Biology of Lung Cancer: Diagnosis and Treatment, *edited by Steven T. Rosen, James L. Mulshine, Frank Cuttitta, and Paul G. Abrams*
38. Pulmonary Vascular Physiology and Pathophysiology, *edited by E. Kenneth Weir and John T. Reeves*
39. Comparative Pulmonary Physiology: Current Concepts, *edited by Stephen C. Wood*
40. Respiratory Physiology: An Analytical Approach, *edited by H. K. Chang and Manuel Paiva*
41. Lung Cell Biology, *edited by Donald Massaro*
42. Heart–Lung Interactions in Health and Disease, *edited by Steven M. Scharf and Sharon S. Cassidy*
43. Clinical Epidemiology of Chronic Obstructive Pulmonary Disease, *edited by Michael J. Hensley and Nicholas A. Saunders*
44. Surgical Pathology of Lung Neoplasms, *edited by Alberto M. Marchevsky*
45. The Lung in Rheumatic Diseases, *edited by Grant W. Cannon and Guy A. Zimmerman*
46. Diagnostic Imaging of the Lung, *edited by Charles E. Putman*
47. Models of Lung Disease: Microscopy and Structural Methods, *edited by Joan Gil*
48. Electron Microscopy of the Lung, *edited by Dean E. Schraufnagel*

49. *Asthma: Its Pathology and Treatment,* edited by Michael A. Kaliner, Peter J. Barnes, and Carl G. A. Persson
50. *Acute Respiratory Failure: Second Edition,* edited by Warren M. Zapol and Francois Lemaire
51. *Lung Disease in the Tropics,* edited by Om P. Sharma
52. *Exercise: Pulmonary Physiology and Pathophysiology,* edited by Brian J. Whipp and Karlman Wasserman
53. *Developmental Neurobiology of Breathing,* edited by Gabriel G. Haddad and Jay P. Farber
54. *Mediators of Pulmonary Inflammation,* edited by Michael A. Bray and Wayne H. Anderson
55. *The Airway Epithelium,* edited by Stephen G. Farmer and Douglas Hay
56. *Physiological Adaptations in Vertebrates: Respiration, Circulation, and Metabolism,* edited by Stephen C. Wood, Roy E. Weber, Alan R. Hargens, and Ronald W. Millard
57. *The Bronchial Circulation,* edited by John Butler
58. *Lung Cancer Differentiation: Implications for Diagnosis and Treatment,* edited by Samuel D. Bernal and Paul J. Hesketh
59. *Pulmonary Complications of Systemic Disease,* edited by John F. Murray
60. *Lung Vascular Injury: Molecular and Cellular Response,* edited by Arnold Johnson and Thomas J. Ferro
61. *Cytokines of the Lung,* edited by Jason Kelley
62. *The Mast Cell in Health and Disease,* edited by Michael A. Kaliner and Dean D. Metcalfe
63. *Pulmonary Disease in the Elderly Patient,* edited by Donald A. Mahler
64. *Cystic Fibrosis,* edited by Pamela B. Davis
65. *Signal Transduction in Lung Cells,* edited by Jerome S. Brody, David M. Center, and Vsevolod A. Tkachuk
66. *Tuberculosis: A Comprehensive International Approach,* edited by Lee B. Reichman and Earl S. Hershfield
67. *Pharmacology of the Respiratory Tract: Experimental and Clinical Research,* edited by K. Fan Chung and Peter J. Barnes
68. *Prevention of Respiratory Diseases,* edited by Albert Hirsch, Marcel Goldberg, Jean-Pierre Martin, and Roland Masse
69. *Pneumocystis carinii Pneumonia: Second Edition, Revised and Expanded,* edited by Peter D. Walzer
70. *Fluid and Solute Transport in the Airspaces of the Lungs,* edited by Richard M. Effros and H. K. Chang
71. *Sleep and Breathing: Second Edition, Revised and Expanded,* edited by Nicholas A. Saunders and Colin E. Sullivan
72. *Airway Secretion: Physiological Bases for the Control of Mucous Hypersecretion,* edited by Tamotsu Takishima and Sanae Shimura
73. *Sarcoidosis and Other Granulomatous Disorders,* edited by D. Geraint James
74. *Epidemiology of Lung Cancer,* edited by Jonathan M. Samet
75. *Pulmonary Embolism,* edited by Mario Morpurgo
76. *Sports and Exercise Medicine,* edited by Stephen C. Wood and Robert C. Roach
77. *Endotoxin and the Lungs,* edited by Kenneth L. Brigham

78. The Mesothelial Cell and Mesothelioma, *edited by Marie-Claude Jaurand and Jean Bignon*
79. Regulation of Breathing: Second Edition, Revised and Expanded, *edited by Jerome A. Dempsey and Allan I. Pack*
80. Pulmonary Fibrosis, *edited by Sem Hin Phan and Roger S. Thrall*
81. Long-Term Oxygen Therapy: Scientific Basis and Clinical Application, *edited by Walter J. O'Donohue, Jr.*
82. Ventral Brainstem Mechanisms and Control of Respiration and Blood Pressure, *edited by C. Ovid Trouth, Richard M. Millis, Heidrun F. Kiwull-Schöne, and Marianne E. Schläfke*
83. A History of Breathing Physiology, *edited by Donald F. Proctor*
84. Surfactant Therapy for Lung Disease, *edited by Bengt Robertson and H. William Taeusch*
85. The Thorax: Second Edition, Revised and Expanded (in three parts), *edited by Charis Roussos*
86. Severe Asthma: Pathogenesis and Clinical Management, *edited by Stanley J. Szefler and Donald Y. M. Leung*
87. Mycobacterium avium–Complex Infection: Progress in Research and Treatment, *edited by Joyce A. Korvick and Constance A. Benson*
88. Alpha 1–Antitrypsin Deficiency: Biology • Pathogenesis • Clinical Manifestations • Therapy, *edited by Ronald G. Crystal*
89. Adhesion Molecules and the Lung, *edited by Peter A. Ward and Joseph C. Fantone*
90. Respiratory Sensation, *edited by Lewis Adams and Abraham Guz*
91. Pulmonary Rehabilitation, *edited by Alfred P. Fishman*
92. Acute Respiratory Failure in Chronic Obstructive Pulmonary Disease, *edited by Jean-Philippe Derenne, William A. Whitelaw, and Thomas Similowski*
93. Environmental Impact on the Airways: From Injury to Repair, *edited by Jacques Chrétien and Daniel Dusser*
94. Inhalation Aerosols: Physical and Biological Basis for Therapy, *edited by Anthony J. Hickey*
95. Tissue Oxygen Deprivation: From Molecular to Integrated Function, *edited by Gabriel G. Haddad and George Lister*
96. The Genetics of Asthma, *edited by Stephen B. Liggett and Deborah A. Meyers*
97. Inhaled Glucocorticoids in Asthma: Mechanisms and Clinical Actions, *edited by Robert P. Schleimer, William W. Busse, and Paul M. O'Byrne*
98. Nitric Oxide and the Lung, *edited by Warren M. Zapol and Kenneth D. Bloch*
99. Primary Pulmonary Hypertension, *edited by Lewis J. Rubin and Stuart Rich*
100. Lung Growth and Development, *edited by John A. McDonald*
101. Parasitic Lung Diseases, *edited by Adel A. F. Mahmoud*
102. Lung Macrophages and Dendritic Cells in Health and Disease, *edited by Mary F. Lipscomb and Stephen W. Russell*
103. Pulmonary and Cardiac Imaging, *edited by Caroline Chiles and Charles E. Putman*
104. Gene Therapy for Diseases of the Lung, *edited by Kenneth L. Brigham*

105. Oxygen, Gene Expression, and Cellular Function, *edited by Linda Biadasz Clerch and Donald J. Massaro*
106. Beta$_2$-Agonists in Asthma Treatment, *edited by Romain Pauwels and Paul M. O'Byrne*
107. Inhalation Delivery of Therapeutic Peptides and Proteins, *edited by Akwete Lex Adjei and Pramod K. Gupta*
108. Asthma in the Elderly, *edited by Robert A. Barbee and John W. Bloom*
109. Treatment of the Hospitalized Cystic Fibrosis Patient, *edited by David M. Orenstein and Robert C. Stern*
110. Asthma and Immunological Diseases in Pregnancy and Early Infancy, *edited by Michael Schatz, Robert S. Zeiger, and Henry N. Claman*
111. Dyspnea, *edited by Donald A. Mahler*
112. Proinflammatory and Antiinflammatory Peptides, *edited by Sami I. Said*
113. Self-Management of Asthma, *edited by Harry Kotses and Andrew Harver*
114. Eicosanoids, Aspirin, and Asthma, *edited by Andrew Szczeklik, Ryszard J. Gryglewski, and John R. Vane*
115. Fatal Asthma, *edited by Albert L. Sheffer*
116. Pulmonary Edema, *edited by Michael A. Matthay and David H. Ingbar*
117. Inflammatory Mechanisms in Asthma, *edited by Stephen T. Holgate and William W. Busse*
118. Physiological Basis of Ventilatory Support, *edited by John J. Marini and Arthur S. Slutsky*
119. Human Immunodeficiency Virus and the Lung, *edited by Mark J. Rosen and James M. Beck*
120. Five-Lipoxygenase Products in Asthma, *edited by Jeffrey M. Drazen, Sven-Erik Dahlén, and Tak H. Lee*
121. Complexity in Structure and Function of the Lung, *edited by Michael P. Hlastala and H. Thomas Robertson*
122. Biology of Lung Cancer, *edited by Madeleine A. Kane and Paul A. Bunn, Jr.*
123. Rhinitis: Mechanisms and Management, *edited by Robert M. Naclerio, Stephen R. Durham, and Niels Mygind*
124. Lung Tumors: Fundamental Biology and Clinical Management, *edited by Christian Brambilla and Elisabeth Brambilla*
125. Interleukin-5: From Molecule to Drug Target for Asthma, *edited by Colin J. Sanderson*
126. Pediatric Asthma, *edited by Shirley Murphy and H. William Kelly*
127. Viral Infections of the Respiratory Tract, *edited by Raphael Dolin and Peter F. Wright*
128. Air Pollutants and the Respiratory Tract, *edited by David L. Swift and W. Michael Foster*
129. Gastroesophageal Reflux Disease and Airway Disease, *edited by Mark R. Stein*
130. Exercise-Induced Asthma, *edited by E. R. McFadden, Jr.*
131. LAM and Other Diseases Characterized by Smooth Muscle Proliferation, *edited by Joel Moss*
132. The Lung at Depth, *edited by Claes E. G. Lundgren and John N. Miller*
133. Regulation of Sleep and Circadian Rhythms, *edited by Fred W. Turek and Phyllis C. Zee*

134. Anticholinergic Agents in the Upper and Lower Airways, *edited by Sheldon L. Spector*

ADDITIONAL VOLUMES IN PREPARATION

Immunotherapy in Asthma, *edited by Jean Bousquet and Hans Yssel*

Control of Breathing in Health and Disease, *edited by Murray D. Altose and Yoshikazu Kawakami*

Chronic Lung Disease of Early Infancy, *edited by Richard D. Bland and Jacqueline J. Coalson*

Diagnostic Pulmonary Pathology, *edited by Philip T. Cagle*

Multimodality Treatment of Lung Cancer, *edited by Arthur T. Skarin*

Cytokines in Pulmonary Infectious Disease, *edited by Steven Nelson and Thomas Martin*

Asthma's Impact on Society: the Social and Economic Burden, *edited by Kevin B. Weiss, A. Sonia Buist, and Sean D. Sullivan*

Asthma and Respiratory Infections, *edited by David P. Skoner*

New and Exploratory Therapeutic Agents for Asthma, *edited by Michael Yeadon and Zuzana Diamant*

Particle–Lung Interactions, *edited by Peter Gehr and Joachim Heyder*

Tuberculosis: A Comprehensive International Approach, Second Edition, *edited by Lee B. Reichman and Earl S. Hershfield*

The opinions expressed in these volumes do not necessarily represent the views of the National Institutes of Health.

ANTICHOLINERGIC AGENTS IN THE UPPER AND LOWER AIRWAYS

Edited by

Sheldon L. Spector

*University of California, Los Angeles, School of Medicine
Los Angeles, California*

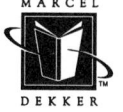

MARCEL DEKKER, INC. NEW YORK · BASEL

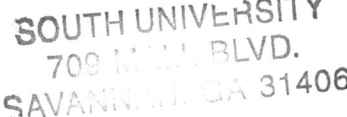

Library of Congress Cataloging-in-Publication Data

Anticholinergic agents in the upper and lower airways / edited by
   Sheldon L. Spector.
      p.   cm. — (Lung biology in health and disease ; 134)
   Includes bibliographical references and indexes.
   ISBN 0-8247-1959-X (alk. paper)
   1. Respiratory organs—Diseases—Chemotherapy.
   2. Parasympatholytic agents.   3. Muscarinic receptors.   4. Asthma—
Chemotherapy.   5. Bronchodilator agents.   I. Spector, Sheldon L.
   [DNLM: 1. Cholinergic Antagonists—pharmacology.   2. Cholinergic
Antagonists—therapeutic use.   3. Bronchodilator Agents—
pharmacology.   4. Bronchodilator Agents—therapeutic use.
5. Respiratory Tract Diseases—drug therapy.   QV 124 A629 1999]
RC735.C47A56   1999
616.2′00461—dc21
DNLM/DLC
for Library of Congress   99-29626
                                                                                                              CIP

This book is printed on acid-free paper.

Headquarters
Marcel Dekker, Inc.
270 Madison Avenue, New York, NY 10016
tel: 212-696-9000; fax: 212-685-4540

Eastern Hemisphere Distribution
Marcel Dekker AG
Hutgasse 4, Postfach 812, CH-4001 Basel, Switzerland
tel: 41-61-261-8482; fax: 41-61-261-8896

World Wide Web
http://www.dekker.com

The publisher offers discounts on this book when ordered in bulk quantities. For more information, write to Special Sales/Professional Marketing at the headquarters address above.

Copyright © 1999 by Marcel Dekker, Inc. All Rights Reserved.

Neither this book nor any part may be reproduced or transmitted in any form or by any means, electronic or mechanical, including photocopying, microfilming, and recording, or by any information storage and retrieval system, without permission in writing from the publisher.

Current printing (last digit):
10 9 8 7 6 5 4 3 2 1

PRINTED IN THE UNITED STATES OF AMERICA

Introduction

Today, allergic reactions such as asthma and rhinitis can be treated by a great number of medications, each with a specific mode of action. Indeed, the last few decades have given clinical physicians impressive arrays of therapeutic approaches, largely based on current understanding of the pathogenesis of the symptoms.

In Chapter 9 of this volume, Kenneth Chapman traces the therapeutic history of one class of drugs—the antimuscarinic bronchodilators—from long before the beginning of the Christian Era. One may then ask, "Why a volume on anticholinergics?" The response to this can be found in the last sentence of Dr. Chapman's chapter. To paraphrase, it says that medications from this class have the same role to play today that they had a century ago, and again, a century before, and again . . . and again.

But meanwhile, the rationale for using these medications has been elucidated. This is true with regard to the relief they give to the asthmatic patient and to the patient who suffers from rhinitis. And so, this volume was conceived to provide and update discussion of the use of anticholinergic medications, either alone or as complements to other therapeutic agents.

Anticholinergic compounds have been used for so long that today few investigators make them the subject of their research. Fortunately, Dr. Spector, the editor of this monograph, identified leaders in the field and invited them to make the unique contributions assembled in this volume. There is no doubt that clinicians will be aided by the discussions the book contains and that patients will benefit from their new understanding.

The Lung Biology in Health and Disease series is proud to present this new and timely contribution.

Claude Lenfant, M.D.
Bethesda, Maryland

Preface

Asthma afflicts 2% to 4% of the U.S. population, and rhinitis afflicts one of every five Americans. Although there are many separate books on the treatment of rhinitis and asthma, it is unusual to find a book that deals with the upper and lower airways in an integrated way, especially with regard to cholinergic mechanisms.

Patients with rhinitis and asthma are heterogeneous with respect to triggers, pathogenesis, and treatment. On the other hand, the upper and lower airways have many things in common, and the stimulus to or treatment of one may very well influence the other. Although the primary aim of this work is to discuss the clinical application of antimuscarinics, chapters are included on the physiological and molecular aspects of anticholinergic therapy in order to provide background for clinical discussion.

In Chapter 1, Drs. Mullol and Baraniuk discuss the concept of hyperresponsiveness and the M_2 and M_3 receptors, which are the predominant muscarinic subtypes in the human respiratory tract. In Chapter 2, Dr. Barnes elaborates on the muscarinic receptors and discusses their interactions with other substances, such as protein kinase C, cytokines, and growth factors, that magnify the effect of these receptors.

Dr. Gross discusses these agents as bronchodilators in Chapter 3. The caliber of resting airways is controlled by bronchomotor tone that involves muscarinic receptors, and reflex bronchospastic mechanisms operate in human airways.

Antimuscarinic drugs also play an important role in the treatment of an acute severe asthmatic attack. The literature on this subject is reviewed by Dr. Garrett in Chapter 4.

Anticholinergic agents also play an important role in the upper airways, not only in the treatment of rhinitis (particularly rhinorrhea), as discussed by Dr. Finn in Chapter 5, but also in the treatment of upper respiratory infections, as discussed by Dr. Spector in Chapter 6.

The concept of combination therapy carries over into many fields in the treatment of rhinitis and asthma. The data regarding beta-agonists combined with antimuscarinics are reviewed in Chapter 7 by Dr. Rennard. And on the horizon is the use of tiotropium bromide, which has interesting characteristics as a bronchodilator with a very long half-life. This has been reviewed by Drs. Witek, Souhrada, Serby, and Disse in Chapter 8.

These discussions are placed in historical perspective in Chapter 9 by Dr. Chapman. Finally, in Chapter 10, some interesting new work regarding the interaction of viruses and the muscarinic receptor is reviewed by Drs. Jacoby and Fryer.

Although such a focused discussion might be expected to be directed toward the subspecialties of allergy and chest medicine, the care of asthmatic patients involves any discipline; physicians in family practice, pediatrics, or internal medicine might very well find this latest information of great interest. The editor sincerely hopes that this comprehensive approach to a specific aspect of the treatment of rhinitis and asthma will be useful to the reader.

I wish to thank not only the contributors, but also Claude Lenfant for his encouragement and his ability to motivate and expedite.

Sheldon L. Spector

Contributors

James N. Baraniuk, M.D.   Associate Professor, Division of Rheumatology, Immunology and Allergy, Georgetown University, Washington, D.C.

Peter J. Barnes, D.M., D.Sc., F.R.C.P.   Professor, Department of Thoracic Medicine, National Heart and Lung Institute, Imperial College, London, England

Kenneth R. Chapman, M.D., M.Sc., F.R.C.P.C., F.A.C.P.   Professor of Medicine, University of Toronto, Toronto, Ontario, Canada

Bernd Disse, M.D., Ph.D.   Head, Therapeutic Area II—Respiratory, Boehringer Ingelheim, Ingelheim, Germany

Albert F. Finn, Jr., M.D.   Clinical Assistant Professor, Departments of Medicine, Microbiology, and Immunology, Medical University of South Carolina, Charleston, South Carolina

Allison D. Fryer, Ph.D. Associate Professor of Physiology, Department of Environmental Health Sciences, Johns Hopkins University, Baltimore, Maryland

Jeffrey E. Garrett, M.D., F.R.A.C.P. Clinical Director, Respiratory Services, Green Lane Hospital, Auckland, New Zealand

Nicholas J. Gross, M.D., Ph.D., F.R.C.P.(Lond), F.A.C.P. Professor, Departments of Medicine and Molecular Biochemistry, Loyola University of Chicago, Chicago, and Attending Physician, Hines VA Hospital, Hines, Illinois

David B. Jacoby, M.D. Head, Pulmonary Drug Discovery, Bristol-Myers Squibb, Princeton, New Jersey

Joaquim Mullol, M.D., Ph.D. Senior Investigator, Fundació Clínic per a la Recerca Biomèdica, Institut d'Investigacions Biomèdiques "August Pi i Sunyer" (IDIBAPS), Barcelona, Catalonia, Spain

Stephen I. Rennard, M.D. Professor of Medicine, Department of Internal Medicine, University of Nebraska Medical Center, Omaha, Nebraska

Charles W. Serby, M.D. Clinical Program Director, Department of Clinical Research, Boehringer Ingelheim Pharmaceuticals, Inc., Ridgefield, Connecticut

Joseph F. Souhrada, M.D., Ph.D. Distinguished Clinical Scientist, Department of Clinical Research—Respiratory, Boehringer Ingelheim Pharmaceuticals, Inc., Ridgefield, and Lecturer in Medicine and Public Health, Yale University School of Medicine, New Haven, Connecticut

Sheldon L. Spector, M.D. Clinical Professor, Department of Medicine, University of California, Los Angeles, School of Medicine, Los Angeles, California

Theodore J. Witek, Jr., Dr.P.H. Therapeutic Area Director, Department of Clinical Research, Boehringer Ingelheim Pharmaceuticals, Inc., Ridgefield, Connecticut, and Research Associate Professor, Department of Pulmonary Medicine, Mount Sinai School of Medicine, New York, New York

Contents

Introduction   Claude Lenfant   *iii*
Preface   *v*
Contributors   *vii*

Part One   BASIC SCIENCE

1. Basics of Muscarinic Physiology   3

Joaquim Mullol and James N. Baraniuk

    I. Introduction   3
    II. Cholinergic Ganglia and Efferent Nerves   4
    III. Pharmacology of Muscarinic Receptors   8
    IV. Muscarinic Receptor Structure   10
    V. M_1 Receptors   13
    VI. M_2 Receptors   14
    VII. M_3 Receptors   16
    VIII. M_4 Receptors   17

	IX.	M_5 Receptors	17
	X.	Physiology of Nasal Cholinergic Reflexes	17
	XI.	Hyperresponsiveness	18
	XII.	Summary	21
		References	22

2. Airway Muscarinic Receptors — 31

Peter J. Barnes

I.	Introduction	31
II.	M_1 Receptors	33
III.	M_2 Receptors	35
IV.	M_3 Receptors	39
V.	M_4 and M_5 Receptors	40
VI.	Clinical Relevance of Muscarinic Receptor Subtypes	40
VII.	Tiotropium Bromide	41
VIII.	Regulation of Muscarinic Receptor Expression	43
	References	49

Part Two APPLIED CLINICAL RESEARCH

3. Anticholinergic Agents as Bronchodilators — 59

Nicholas J. Gross

I.	Rationale for Use of Anticholinergic Agents	59
II.	Cholinergic Muscarinic Receptors in Airways	60
III.	Available and Experimental Anticholinergic Agents	62
IV.	Features of Anticholinergic Bronchodilator Actions	63
V.	Clinical Actions	65
VI.	Side Effects	69
	References	69

4. Anticholinergic Drug Therapy in the Management of Acute Severe Asthma — 73

Jeffrey E. Garrett

I.	Introduction	73
II.	What Is the Optimal Dose of Ipratropium Bromide in Acute Severe Asthma?	75
III.	Does Inhaled Ipratropium Bromide Augment the Effect of Beta-Agonist Therapy?	75

Contents   xi

	IV.	Does Inhaled Ipratropium Bromide Contribute Anything to Maximally Employed Beta-Agonist Therapy?	77
	V.	Does Ipratropium Bromide Contribute to Improvements in Clinical Outcomes?	78
	VI.	Is There a Pharmacoeconomic Argument for the Use of Inhaled Ipratropium Bromide in Acute Asthma?	80
	VII.	Are There Patient Subgroups Who Derive Particular Benefit from Anticholinergic Therapy?	80
	VIII.	Summary	82
		References	82

5. Use of Anticholinergics in Perennial Rhinitis   87

Albert F. Finn, Jr.

	I.	Introduction	87
	II.	Pathophysiology of Perennial Rhinitis	89
	III.	Cholinergic Mechanisms in Perennial Rhinitis	91
	IV.	Anticholinergic Agents in Perennial and Nonallergic Rhinitis	93
	V.	Summary	96
		References	96

6. Pathogenesis and Treatment of Upper Respiratory Infections   101

Sheldon L. Spector

	I.	Introduction	101
	II.	Pathogenesis and Epidemiology	102
	III.	Management of the Common Cold	104
	IV.	Prevention	109
	V.	Conclusion	110
		References	111

7. Anticholinergics in Combination Bronchodilator Therapy in COPD   119

Stephen I. Rennard

	I.	Introduction	119
	II.	Bronchodilators and Expiratory Airflow Limitation	120
	III.	Rationale for Combined Bronchodilator Therapy	122

IV.	Conclusion	129
	References	130

8. Tiotropium (Ba 679): Pharmacology and Early Clinical Observations — 137

Theodore J. Witek, Jr., Joseph F. Souhrada, Charles W. Serby, and Bernd Disse

I.	Introduction	137
II.	Pharmacology	138
III.	Human Pharmacology and Early Clinical Trials	142
IV.	Potential Role in Clinical Practice	147
V.	Summary and Conclusions	149
	References	150

Part Three TOPICS OF SPECIAL INTEREST

9. Historical Aspects of Medicinal Uses of Antimuscarinics — 155

Kenneth R. Chapman

I.	Introduction	155
II.	*Datura*	156
III.	Psychotropic Uses of Antimuscarinic Botanicals	157
IV.	Anticholinergic Bronchodilators	160
V.	Antimuscarinic Therapy—Early Mechanistic Studies	163
VI.	Efficacy of Asthma Cigarettes	165
VII.	Modern Quaternary Antimuscarinics	166
VIII.	The Future of Antimuscarinic Bronchodilator Therapy	167
IX.	Summary	167
	References	167

10. Interaction of Virus with the Muscarinic Receptor — 171

David B. Jacoby and Allison D. Fryer

I.	Introduction	171
II.	Virus-Induced Parasympathetic Hyperresponsiveness	173
III.	Conclusion	181
	References	182

Author Index	*189*
Subject Index	*209*

Part One

BASIC SCIENCE

1

Basics of Muscarinic Physiology

JOAQUIM MULLOL

Institut d'Investigacions Biomèdiques
"August Pi i Sunyer" (IDIBAPS)
Barcelona, Catalonia, Spain

JAMES N. BARANIUK

Georgetown University
Washington, D.C.

I. Introduction

Anticholinergic drugs have utility-regulating smooth muscle tone and glandular secretion in chronic obstructive pulmonary disease, asthma, allergic rhinitis, and sinusitis. Parasympathetic cholinergic reflexes are the most potent tonically active regulators of bronchoconstriction and submucosal gland exocytosis and secretion in the airways. The actions of acetylcholine (ACh) on end organs and the release of ACh from postganglionic neurons are regulated by specific muscarinic receptor subtypes. Four receptors have been defined by pharmacologic ligand binding studies (M_1 to M_4), while five (and possibly seven) muscarinic receptor genes (m_1 to m_5) have been cloned (1–3). ACh is synthesized in peripheral nerves by choline acetyltransferase and stored in secretory vesicles. ACh's actions are limited by degradation by acetylcholinesterase, an enzyme that is widely expressed on airway cells.

II. Cholinergic Ganglia and Efferent Nerves

Preganglionic vagal efferent fibers originate in the dorsal motor nucleus of the 10th nerve in the brainstem and innervate laryngeal and tracheobronchial parasympathetic ganglia. Nasal cavity, ethmoid sinus, and anterior nasopharyngeal parasympathetic innervation are derived from preganglionic seventh nerve motor fibers that originate in the superior salivatory nucleus and pass through the Vidian canal to synapse in the sphenopalatine ganglion. Brainstem parasympathetic nuclei are capable of inducing independent nasal, laryngeal, and tracheobronchial efferent responses. This contrasts with the generalized, "all-or-nothing" response of the sympathetic nervous system. Additional glossopharyngeal, vagal, and spinal accessory motor neurons innervate pharyngeal, laryngeal, and upper esophageal striated muscle, and participate in the gag reflex.

Tracheobronchial ganglia contain a half dozen to a score of individual neuron cell bodies. In ferret trachea, large-diameter, centrally located ganglion cell bodies contain ACh; smaller-diameter cell bodies contain vasoactive intestinal peptide (VIP) and nitric oxide synthase (NOS) (4). In this species, these two postganglionic populations may regulate cholinergic smooth muscle contraction and glandular exocytosis and noncholinergic vasodilatation. The situation in human ganglia may be more complex and may depend upon the inflammatory state of the airways, level of expression of NOS (5), and the colocalization of other VIP-like neurotransmitters such as peptide with histidine at the N-terminal and methionine at the C-terminal (PHM) (6,7). Ganglion cells have "plasticity," since they can alter their neurotransmitter phenotype. For example, neuropeptide tyrosine (NPY) can be induced after heart-lung transplant (8). It remains undetermined if there are analogous changes during airway inflammatory diseases such as asthma.

ACh released from preganglionic neurons binds to the extracellular domains of nicotinic N_2 receptors (N_1 = skeletal muscle type; N_2 = ganglionic type) of postganglionic neurons (Fig. 1). Nicotinic receptors are ligand-gated Na^+ channels. N_2 receptors are preferentially activated by 1,1-dimethyl-4-phenylpiperazinium (DMPP) and inhibited by classical ganglion blockers such as hexamethonium and chlorisondamine. Postganglionic M_1 receptors facilitate depolarization and cholinergic neurotransmission (9).

Parasympathetic ganglia are also innervated by nociceptive sensory neurons that contain substance P (SP), neurokinin A (NKA), calcitonin gene-related peptide (CGRP), and possibly other neurotransmitters that may act upon "excitatory" autoreceptors to stimulate postganglionic cell depolariza-

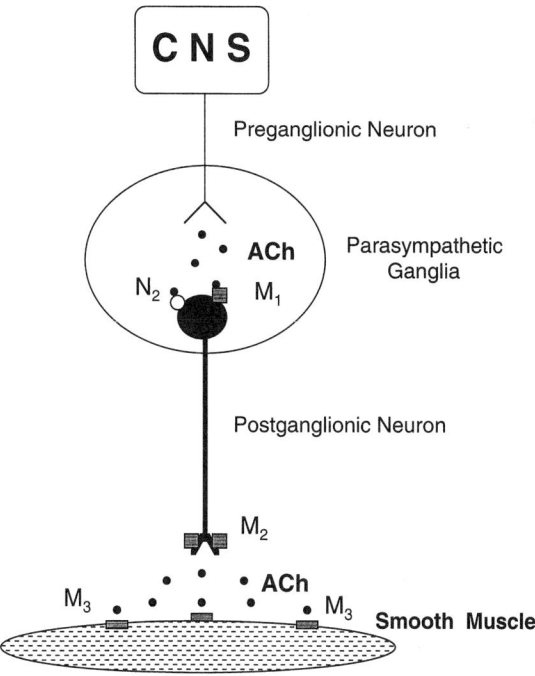

Figure 1 Parasympathetic innervation. Preganglionic fibers innervate parabronchial ganglionic cells and release acetylcholine (ACh) that acts on nicotinic N_2 receptor ion channels and muscarinic M_1 receptors to cause postganglionic cell depolarization. The postganglionic fibers release ACh that acts on M_3 receptors on muscle and glands. M_2 receptors on smooth muscle cells and postganglionic fiber endings may have regulatory function.

tion (Fig. 2) (1,2,6,7). Neurokinin type 3 subtype receptors (NK_3-R, neurokinin B-preferring receptor) mediate the generation of slow excitatory postsynaptic potentials (EPSP) on parasympathetic nerves, while NK-1 receptors (SP-preferring) may have an analogous function on sympathetic nerves. Prostaglandins and leukotrienes may promote the actions of excitatory autoreceptors by reducing the threshold for depolarization. Sympathetic neurons that innervate parasympathetic ganglia release norepinephrine and probably neuropeptide Y (NPY), which may act upon "inhibitory" α_2-adrenergic or NPY Y_2 autoreceptors to decrease the frequency of postganglion cell depolarization (1). Circulating epinephrine may act upon β_2-adrenergic autoreceptors. Other

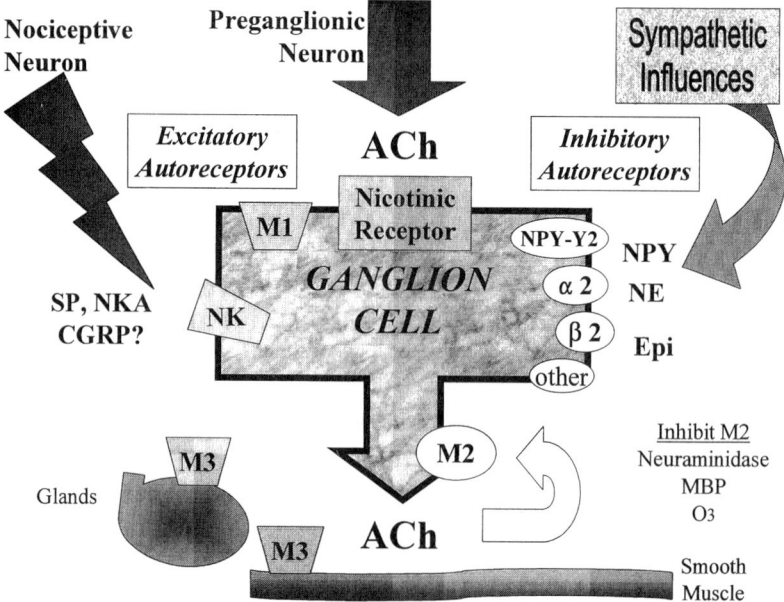

Figure 2 Ganglion cell regulation. Postganglionic cells are innervated by parasympathetic preganglionic, sensory, and sympathetic neurons. Parasympathetic preganglionic cells release ACh that activates nicotinic N_2 receptors to depolarize the ganglion cell. M_1 receptors promote this function. Tachykinins released from nociceptive sensory neurons may activate the ganglion cell via excitatory NK-3 autoreceptors. Inhibitory autoreceptors such as α_2- and β_2-adrenergic, NPY Y_2, $GABA_B$, and μ-opioid receptors may be activated by sympathetic neurotransmitters, humoral, and other mediators to suppress ganglion depolarization. M_2 autoreceptors on postganglionic dendrites may reduce ACh release.

inhibitory autoreceptors include muscarinic M_2, $GABA_B$, histamine H_3, and μ-opioid receptors (1,2). These inhibitory autoreceptors may open a potassium channel that hyperpolarizes the ganglion, making it more difficult to induce depolarization. Because of this "decision-making" function, the ganglion cell can be thought of as an electrical "filter" that integrates incoming inhibitory and excitatory signals to "decide" its own rate of depolarization, subsequent ACh release, and tonic cholinergic bronchoconstrictor and glandular secretion tone.

VIP and PHM may influence postganglionic ACh release (10). ACh is released at low nerve impulse frequency rates, while at high rates, ACh and

VIP are released. VIP may augment the postsynaptic acetylcholine-induced secretory response in glands (e.g., cat salivary glands [11]), but may also have presynaptic inhibitory effects to limit neuropeptide release.

Postganglionic cholinergic fibers innervate glands and some vessels in the nasal, pharyngeal, laryngeal, and tracheobronchial mucosa (12–14). In bronchi, these neurons are most dense in the proximal airways, with decreasing densities in the smaller, more distal bronchi and bronchioles, and are essentially nonexistent in the alveoli (15–17). Submucosal smooth muscle and glands are densely innervated, while bronchial epithelium and vessels have very little cholinergic innervation.

VIP nerve fibers innervate smooth muscle, glands, and some vessels (6,7,14). VIP binding sites are present on epithelium, glands, and vessels, suggesting roles in secretion and vasodilatation. In vitro, VIP stimulates glandular secretion in many models but in human bronchial explants inhibits mucous secretion (18,19). Anti-VIP antibodies may play a pathological role in some cases of chronic bronchitis (19). An absence of VIP nerve fibers has been described in status asthmaticus (20) and cystic fibrosis (21). Increased VIP nerve fiber density has been demonstrated in vasomotor rhinitis (chronic cholinergic rhinitis) (22). In vivo, VIP may be more active as a vasodilator than as a secretogogue since atropine blocks essentially all gland secretion but only partially blocks neurogenically induced blood flow (11,23).

Autoradiographic radioligand binding studies indicate that muscarinic receptors are located on airway smooth muscle, submucosal glands, parasympathetic ganglia, and nerve bundles (Table 1) (24–29). There is little binding to epithelium and vessels. In human lung, muscarinic receptors are distributed over both proximal and distal airways and are present in alveoli. Only M_1, M_2, and M_3 receptors have been identified in human airways (30). In bronchial smooth muscle, M_2 and M_3 receptors have been identified (31). Epithelial cells express strong signals for m_3 receptor mRNA by in situ hybridization, but the density of M_3 binding sites is relatively weak, suggesting rapid receptor protein turnover. M_1 receptors are localized to parasympathetic ganglia with M_2 receptors in their peripheral processes (32). Bronchial endothelial cells express M_3 receptors. Alveolar walls express M_1 receptors. mRNA, immunoreactive protein, and binding sites corresponding to M_4 and M_5 receptors have not been identified in human airways.

Muscarinic receptors are expressed in the developing respiratory tract, but only weak bronchoconstrictor responses are generated. This may be the result of delayed G-protein expression or other intracellular events (33).

In the nasal mucosa, M_3 and M_1 receptors are found on glands, with lower levels in epithelial cells, and endothelial cells of arterioles, arteriovenous

Table 1 Autoradiographic Localization of Muscarinic Receptors in Human Nasal and Tracheobronchial Airways

Subtype	Localization	Function
M_1	Parasympathetic ganglia	Facilitate neurotransmission
	Nasal submucosal glands	Exocytosis?
	Alveolar walls	?
M_2	Postganglionic cholinergic nerves	Inhibit ACh release
	Airway smooth muscle	Inhibit adenylyl cyclase and antagonize adrenergic bronchodilation
	Sympathetic nerves	Inhibit norepinephrine release
M_3	Airway smooth muscle	Contraction
	Submucosal glands	Exocytosis
	Goblet cells?	Exocytosis
	Epithelial cells	Increased ciliary beat frequency?
	Endothelial cells	Release of nitric oxide and vasodilation
M_4	Alveolar walls[a]	?
	Airway smooth muscle[a]	?
	Postganglionic cholinergic nerves	Inhibit ACh release

[a]Rabbit only.

anastomoses, capacitance vessels, and venous sinusoids (29,34). M_3 receptors predominate by a 2:1 ratio.

III. Pharmacology of Muscarinic Receptors

The muscarinic receptor family was discovered by the binding of the alkaloid muscarine derived from the mushroom Amanita muscaria. In 1914, Dale demonstrated that ACh induced two separate responses that could be mimicked by either nicotine or muscarine (35). The muscarinic effect could be antagonized by atropine. It took another 70 years to further subdivide these muscarinic effects by using selective antagonists and molecular cloning.

Although five muscarinic receptor genes (m1 to m5) have been cloned, only four of these (M_1 to M_4) have been defined by pharmacological means (2,3,36–38). Currently available agonists and antagonists do not have sufficient selectivity to absolutely discriminate between receptor subtypes (Table 2). Pirenzepine, the first selective antagonist, was used to define the M_1 muscarinic receptor subtype. Pirenzepine, gallamine and AF DX-116 (M_2), 4-DAMP

Table 2 Pharmacology, Mechanism of Action, Distribution, and Function of Muscarinic Receptor Subtypes in the Airways

	M_1	M_2	M_3	M_4	M_5
Selective agonists	McN-A343 Pilocarpine L-689,660	Betanechol Pilocarpine	L-689,660	McN-A343	?
Selective antagonists	Pirenzepine Telenzepine 4-DAMP	Methoctramine AFDX-116 Himbascine Gallamine	4-DAMP Hexahydrosiladifenidol Zamifenacin	Methoctramine Himbascine	?
G protein	G_q	G_i	G_q	G_i	G_q?
Intracellular messenger	IP_3/DAG	cAMP/K^+ channels	IP_3/DAG	cAMP	IP_3/DAG?
Airway distribution	Cholinergic ganglia Alveolar walls Submucosal glands	Cholinergic nerves Smooth muscle	Smooth muscle Submucosal glands Blood vessels (nose)	(Not found in humans)	?
Airway function	Facilitation of neurotransmission Glandular secretion (nose)	Inhibition of neurotransmission (autoreceptor)	Smooth muscle contraction Glandular secretion Vasodilation (nose)	Regulation of chloride secretion?	?

(M_3) and himbascine (M_2 and M_4) have been used to define particular muscarinic functions, but this task is complex since multiple subtypes may be present on end organs, and the antagonists have only partial selectivity. For example, in guinea pig ileal smooth muscle, M_2 receptors account for approximately 80% of the total binding capacity, yet M_3 receptor stimulation (20% of tissue muscarinic receptors) accounts for essentially all the cholinergically induced contraction (3). No agonists or antagonists have been identified for M_5 receptors (38).

IV. Muscarinic Receptor Structure

The five cloned muscarinic receptors belong to the rhodopsin family of G-protein-related receptors that bind sensory molecules (light, odorants), biogenic amines (muscarinic, dopamine, epinephrine, norepinephrine, histamine, serotonin), glycoprotein hormones (including TRH and FSH), neuropeptides and peptide hormones (substance P, bradykinin, gastrin-releasing peptide, cholecystokinin, many others), IL8, and other mediators (39,40). These proteins have a characteristic structure with glycosylated extracellular NH_2 terminal, seven transmembrane regions (Tm_1 to Tm_7), three extracellular loops (E_1 to E_3), three intracellular or cytoplasmic loops (C_1 to C_3), and an intracellular COOH tail (Fig. 3).

The seven transmembrane regions are amphipathic helical cylinders that are stacked parallel to each other as they span the membrane. The intra- and extracellular loops are like tethers that group the cylinders together. Two cysteines in E_1 and E_2 form a disulfide bond that constrains the side-by-side orientation of Tm_2, Tm_3, Tm_4, and Tm_5 (41). Amino acid interactions between adjacent cylinders determine the spacing of the cylinders. Amino acids that project from the cylinders into the oblong space between the seven cylinders form the ACh binding pocket. These interacting amino acids generate a "charged pit" within the otherwise hydrophobic helices and membrane lipid environment and determine the specificity and avidity of ligand binding. The amino acids defining the ligand-binding sites differ among subtypes (42–45). Understanding of the chemistry of these interactions will lead to the development of more selective and effective agonist and antagonist compounds. A full explanation of this fascinating insight into receptor function is beyond the scope of this review. Only selective principles will be discussed.

The Tm helices are not completely cylindrical. Prolines in Tm_5, Tm_6, and Tm_7 are highly conserved among these receptors. Proline disrupts, or "breaks," α-helices, and may warp Tm_5, Tm_6, and Tm_7, perhaps allowing

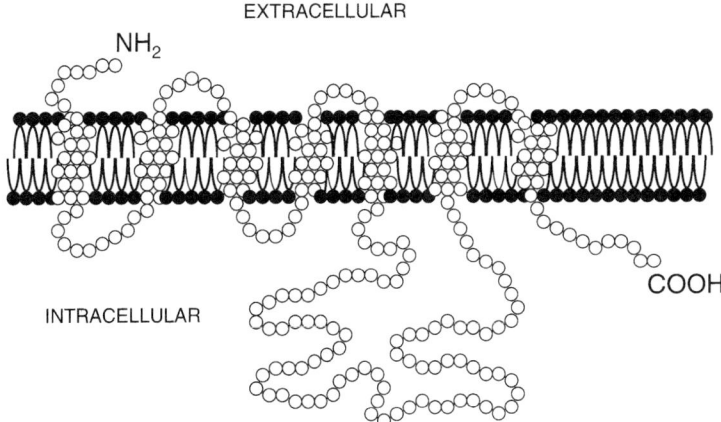

Figure 3 Prototypic structure of seven transmembrane muscarinic receptors. The extracellular amino terminal, seven transmembrane regions, three extracellular loops, three intracellular loops, and an intracellular carboxyterminal are shown. The extracellular domains have carbohydrate side chains that may be essential for receptor function. The third intracellular domain is the G-protein binding region.

them to stack next to each other within the membrane like stackable chairs. Point mutations of each of these prolines reduce the membrane expression of these receptors, suggesting that these bends are essential for receptor packaging or transport into the membrane. Substitution of proline to alanine reduces the ability of carbachol to induce signal transduction but does not alter ligand binding, suggesting that the transmembrane regions have two functions: ligand binding in the portions of the helices near the extracellular surface, and transduction of ligand binding-induced conformation changes to the intracellular portions of the receptor (39). Other key amino acids that contribute to the essential tertiary structure are shared by other amine receptors such as α- and β-adrenergic receptor subtypes (19).

Each C_3 has a highly unique sequence. This is the region with the least homology between muscarinic receptor subtypes (40). The M_3 receptor has an amphipathic α-helix that is essential for G-protein interaction. Mutations that alter the C_3 helical structure prevent G-protein activation (46). The precise G-proteins that associate with each muscarinic receptor are still being defined, but it appears that M_1, M_3, and M_5 receptors bind with G_q proteins that activate phospholipase C, while M_2 and M_4 receptors bind G_i that inhibit adenylyl cyclase (Table 2) (2,3,40,47). The COOH tails contain phosphorylation sites that may regulate the binding of G-proteins or lead to receptor desensitization or tachyphylaxis (39).

These data suggest that the ligand-binding site consists of a pocket formed by adjacent surfaces of the transmembrane helices, that ligand binding induces conformational rotations or shifts in position of these helices relative to each other, and that these conformational changes are translated to the third intracellular (C3) G-protein-binding region, or C-terminal tail to promote G-protein binding. While the ligand-binding regions of the five muscarinic receptors are relatively highly conserved, the intracytoplasmic C_3 loop and C terminal are very divergent, suggesting that differences in G-protein binding specificities are the principal differences between the receptor subtypes. The functions of each receptor subtype will depend upon the actions of these G-proteins and their signaling pathways within different cell types. M_1, M_3, and possibly M_5 receptors are linked to G_q proteins that stimulate the opening of Ca^{2+} channels and the release of arachidonic acid, phosphatidic acid, and inositol-tris-phosphate (IP_3) plus diacylglycerol (DAG) by the actions of phospholipase A_2, D, and C_β, respectively (Fig. 4) (40). These activate calcium chan-

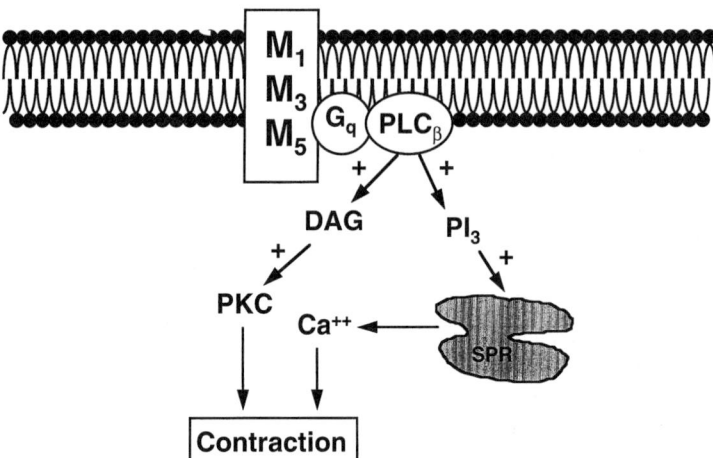

Figure 4 M_1, M_3, and probably M_5 receptors are linked to G_q protein that activates phospholipases. PLC_β may be of preeminent importance and lead to release of phosphoinositol (PI_3) and diacylglycerol (DAG). PI_3 opens Ca^{2+} channels in smooth endoplasmic reticulum (SPR), leading to an increase in intracellular calcium, while DAG stimulates phosphokinase C (PKC) activation. These actions lead to smooth muscle contraction.

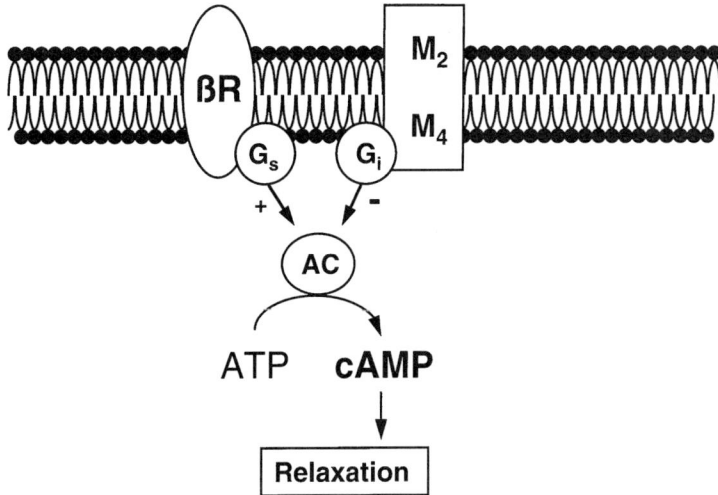

Figure 5 M_2 and possibly M_4 receptors are linked to G_i proteins that inhibit adenylyl cyclase (AC) and reduce intracellular cAMP levels. This promotes smooth muscle contraction. This system antagonizes the cAMP formation induced by β_2-adrenergic receptors and their G_S proteins that stimulate AC activity.

nels and increase intracellular calcium concentrations. M_2 and M_4 receptors are linked to inhibitor G-proteins that decrease the activities of adenylyl cyclase and phospholipase C_β (Fig. 5) (48).

Agonist binding to muscarinic receptors leads to phosphorylation of the C_3 and/or C-terminal tail with functional downregulation of the receptor. This represents homologous desensitization since binding of the cholinergic agonist leads to downregulation. In contrast, activation of β_2-adrenergic receptors may lead to phosphorylation and inactivation of muscarinic receptors (heterologous desensitization) (40).

V. M_1 Receptors

M_1 receptors are most concentrated in cerebral cortex and neural ganglia. In the lungs, M_1 receptors and m_1 mRNA have been demonstrated by radioligand binding studies, Northern blotting, and in situ hybridization in human alveoli and by autoradiography in human nasal mucosa (25,26,29,31). The significance of the alveolar receptors is unclear, since this tissue is not innervated by cholinergic nerves. M_1 receptors predominate in neuronal tissues and are present in parasympathetic (26,28) and sympathetic peripheral neurons (1). These receptors may be functionally important, since pirenzepine, an M_1 antagonist, inhibits the bronchoconstriction induced by electrical vagus nerve stimulation in vitro (49,50) and by inhalation of SO_2 (51), an agent thought to activate nociceptive sensory nerves that recruit parasympathetic bronchoconstrictor reflexes. Pirenzepine does not block the effects of inhaled methacholine. Although M_1 binding sites have been noted on submucosal glands in the bronchial and nasal mucosae, pirenzepine has no effect on cholinergic glandular secretion (26,29,52,53). The identity of these glandular receptors has not been confirmed at the mRNA level, as m_1 mRNA has not been localized to these sites (26).

Nicotinic receptors lead to rapid depolarization and are responsible for transmission of preganglionic signals to the postganglionic neuron. M_1 receptors may facilitate this action by closing potassium channels, resulting in a slow depolarization of ganglion cells.

M_1 receptors can activate both G_{qa} and G_{11a} to initiate phosphoinositol metabolism (2).

VI. M_2 Receptors

M_2 receptors regulate cholinergic ganglion and bronchial smooth muscle function. M_2 receptors are coupled to a pertussis toxin-sensitive G_i protein which inhibits adenylyl cyclase and decreases intracellular cAMP levels (40). Alterations in M_2 receptor functions may lead to cholinergic hyperresponsiveness. M_2 receptors are present in highest density in the heart.

A. Smooth Muscle

M_2 binding sites and m_2 mRNA have been demonstrated in cultured human tracheal smooth muscle cells and airway smooth muscle (54,55). M_2 receptor binding with inhibition of adenylyl cyclase does not alter smooth muscle contraction. However, M_2 receptor activation antagonizes the effects of β_2-adrenergic receptor stimulation and leads to bronchoconstriction, since the β_2-adrenoceptor effects are mediated by stimulation of adenylyl cyclase and increased cAMP production (Fig. 5). Thus, in the presence of high sympathetic tone, parasympathetic cholinergic reflexes would lead to relative bronchoconstriction by activating M_3 receptors (smooth muscle contraction) and M_2 receptors (antagonism of β_2-receptor-induced bronchodilation). High parasympathetic tone would limit the bronchodilator efficacy of β_2-adrenergic agonists.

M_2 receptor stimulation does not appear to affect PGE_1- or PGE_2-induced cAMP formation, suggesting that these are coupled to different adenylyl cyclase isoforms (56). Under certain circumstances, M_2 function is dependent on cyclooxygenase activity. M_2 receptors are sometimes also linked to a pertussis toxin-sensitive G-protein that may activate an ion channel to induce smooth muscle contraction (2,3).

B. Ganglionic Autoreceptors

"Inhibitory" M_2 autoreceptors are present and active in H. sapiens and other species (58). M_2 agonists decrease the release of ACh from parasympathetic ganglia in guinea pig trachea (57–60). Conversely, methoctramine, an M_2 antagonist, increases ACh release and contributes to bronchial hyperresponsiveness (61,62). M_1 and M_3 antagonists have no effect. Pilocarpine, an M_2 agonist, inhibits SO_2-induced bronchoconstriction in humans in vivo (63). Pilocarpine can inhibit electrical nerve stimulation-mediated bronchial smooth muscle contraction but has no effect on ACh-induced contraction. This effect of pilocarpine is blocked by the M_2 antagonist gallamine, suggesting that M_2 receptors on postganglionic cholinergic nerves reduce cholinergic neurotransmission (57). M_2 receptors may also inhibit norepinephrine release from sympathetic nerves (64).

Inhibitory M_2 autoreceptors on ganglion cells may be modified in disease states. Influenza infection of guinea pigs can increase bronchial responses to methacholine. The neuraminidase of the influenza virus is capable of cleaving sialic acid residues from M_2 receptors, thereby inactivating the receptors (65,66). This mechanism could contribute to some cases of postviral bronchospasm. Neuronal M_2 dysfunction is also present in allergen challenge models (65,67) and human asthma (63,68).

Allergic reactions are characterized by eosinophilia and release of eosinophil cationic proteins. Eosinophils are attracted to neurons in airway walls (69). Inhibition of eosinophil chemoattraction using antibodies to IL-5 or VLA-4 maintains M_2-autoreceptor function (62,70,71). Eosinophil major basic protein (MBP) and peroxidase (EPO), but not eosinophil cationic protein (ECP) or eosinophil-derived neurotoxin (EDN), can selectively bind and inactivate M_2 receptors, and lead to ganglionic dysfunction (72). Heparin can antagonize MBP-M_2 binding and reverse hyperresponsiveness to vagal nerve stimulation indicating that eosinophil protein-M_2 receptor interactions are likely to play a role in allergic asthma (73,74).

Ozone may also alter M_2 receptor function (75). Inhalation of O_3 for 8 weeks by pathogen-free guinea pigs induces (1) cholinergic hyperresponsiveness, (2) loss of the ability of M_2-receptor agonists to attenuate cholinergic reflex-mediated bronchoconstriction, and (3) the development of a requirement for prostaglandins for proper functioning of M_2 receptors (76). The mechanism of the prostaglandin dependency is unclear. Dependence upon prostaglandins for autoreceptor function is of interest, since some asthmatic and rhinitis/sinusitis patients have aspirin sensitivity. Blockade of cyclo-oxygenase leads to decreased prostaglandin synthesis and shunting of arachidonic acid toward leukotriene formation, which leads to severe, acute bronchospasm or rhinitis (77).

The combination of M_2 autoreceptor dysfunction plus β_2-adrenergic antagonists could be a very dangerous situation since both the inhibitory influences of epinephrine or norepinephrine and M_2 autoreceptors on ganglion cell transmission would be missing. β_2-Adrenoceptors on smooth muscle cells would also be blocked, again promoting bronchoconstriction.

M_2 receptors are absent from human alveoli and nasal mucosa (29,31,54).

VII. M_3 Receptors

M_3 receptors mediate cholinergic bronchoconstriction and glandular secretion in the human respiratory tract (1,3). M_3 receptor stimulation activates a pertussis toxin insensitive G_q protein that activates phospholipase C (PLC) to release inositol (1,4,5)-trisphosphate (IP_3) and diacylglycerol (DAG) (Fig. 4) (3,38,40,48,78,79). IP_3 releases calcium from intracellular stores, while DAG activates protein kinase C (PKC) (80). The two actions lead to smooth muscle contraction in airway, gastrointestinal, urinary bladder, vascular, and other tissues. Other functions include release of endothelium-dependent relaxing factor, tracheal epithelium-derived relaxing factor, stimulation of guinea pig ileal electrolyte secretion, and rapid induction of E-cadherin by a small-cell lung carcinoma cell line (3,81).

M_3 binding sites and m_3 mRNA are distributed throughout the large and small airways and are localized in high concentration to smooth muscle and submucosal gland cells, where their function is to induce smooth muscle contraction and exocytosis, respectively (25,26,29,53,54). M_3-selective antagonists inhibit cholinergically induced smooth muscle contraction and exocytosis from human tracheobronchial and nasal glands (3,52,54). M_3 receptors are expressed in lower densities on nasal and bronchial epithelium and endothelium, where they are thought to contribute to goblet cell secretion, ion and water transport, and vasodilatation (82,83).

Atropine (84) and ipratropium bromide are nonselective cholinergic antagonists that inhibit M_3-mediated bronchoconstriction and glandular secretion and M_2-mediated neural autoregulation. Newer M_3-selective antagonists such as darifenacin (UK-88,525) and revatropate (UK-112,116) may offer advantages by blocking M_3-mediated bronchial smooth muscle contraction and glandular exocytosis without interfering with M_2 inhibitory autoreceptor mechanisms (85).

VIII. M_4 Receptors

M_4 receptors and m_4 mRNA have been identified in rabbit lung. In situ hybridization localizes it to alveolar walls and bronchial smooth muscle (54,86). The function of these receptors is not known. M_4 receptors have also been postulated to modulate postganglionic cholinergic nerves in guinea pig trachea (30,31,87). m_4 mRNA has not been identified in human bronchial mucosa.

IX. M_5 Receptors

Selective ligands for M_5 receptors have not been developed. m_5 mRNA does not appear to be present in human respiratory tissues (1,30,31).

X. Physiology of Nasal Cholinergic Reflexes

Parasympathetically released acetylcholine is paramount in stimulating submucosal gland secretion in human nasal mucosa (13,14,88). About 55% of the muscarinic receptors are of the M_3 type, while the remainder are M_1 (29). M_1 binding sites are present on epithelium and submucosal glands. M_3 receptors and m_3 mRNA have been identified by autoradiography (15) and in situ hybridization (89), respectively, on the epithelium, submucosal glands, and endothelium. M_2 binding sites are apparently not present in human nasal mucosa. M_4 sites were not examined. Methacholine stimulates both serous and mucous cell exocytosis, an effect that is inhibited by M_3 antagonists, and weakly inhibited by M_1 antagonists in human nasal mucosa (53). M_1 and M_3 receptors may promote ciliary motility (90).

In vivo, cholinergic reflexes act upon resistance vessels to increase superficial blood flow, but there is little effect on capacitance vessels (sinusoids) that control mucosal thickness or postcapillary venules that are the site of vascular permeability (11). M_3 receptors on bronchial, and possibly nasal, endothelial cells may participate in these vasodilatory reflexes (34). Although small amounts of plasma proteins such as albumin and IgG are released in response to methacholine, they do not significantly contribute to secretion production (13). These plasma macromolecules may (1) enter gland ducts and acini from the interstitium by diffusion between acinar cells to be extruded along with glandular macromolecules in mucus, (2) leak from post-capillary venules after activation of M_3 receptors on endothelial cells, or (3) exit fenestrated capillaries when vasodilator reflexes increase the blood pressure transmitted to these readily permeable vessels.

Stimulation of nasal nociceptive sensory nerves by cold dry air, capsaicin, histamine, bradykinin or allergic reactions recruits parasympathetic reflexes (13,14,23). These reflexes are the most important mechanism regulating glandular serous and mucous cell exocytosis, a finding clearly demonstrated in unilateral provocation models. For example, unilateral histamine provocation leads to the direct activation of H_1 receptors on vessels to stimulate arterial dilation, sinusoidal filling with obstruction to nasal airflow, and vascular permeability with the secretion of a fluid enriched by albumin, IgG, and other plasma proteins (13,14). Nociceptive sensory nerves are stimulated to transmit sensations of itch and trigger protective reflexes including sneezing. Bilateral, cholinergic reflexes are recruited that stimulate glandular secretion of mucous cell mucoglycoproteins and serous cell lysozyme, lactoferrin, secretory IgA, and other nonspecific antimicrobial factors. The noncholinergic component of the reflex-mediated nasal obstruction has not been quantified.

The muscarinic antagonists atropine and ipratropium bromide effectively reduce glandular secretion and ''dry'' the mucosa, but have no effect on sneezing or vascular congestion (91). Selective M_3 receptor antagonists may have clinical utility in rhinitis, where parasympathetic glandular secretion is a significant cause of patient discomfort. However, reductions in glandular secretion volume could reduce the amounts of serous cell–derived antimicrobial and lubricating proteins on the mucosal surface and lead to drying of the surface, irritation, and sensory nerve stimulation. Use of cholinergic antagonists in asthma is discussed elsewhere in this text.

XI. Hyperresponsiveness

Cholinergic tone and hyperresponsiveness to methacholine are characteristic findings in asthma (bronchoconstriction) and rhinitis (glandular secretion), but the molecular mechanisms remain elusive (1,92–95). These effects may be due to an increase in the contractile response of bronchial smooth muscle to cholinergic agonists. M_3 receptors have the predominant effect of inducing smooth muscle contraction while M_2 receptors may have no direct effect on smooth muscle contraction in human airways. However, there is no evidence to indicate that alterations in muscarinic receptor density, affinity, expression, signal coupling and transduction, or phosphoinositol turnover exist in asthmatic or rhinitis tissues (96–101).

M_2 receptors on bronchial smooth muscle cells may interfere with β_2-agonist-mediated bronchodilation and so promote bronchoconstriction. Comparisons of the in vitro isoproterenol-induced relaxation dose-response curves for human airway strips that had been precontracted with either carbachol or histamine suggest that carbachol treatment interferes with β_2-receptor-mediated relaxation (102). In contrast, the M_2 antagonist AFX-116 increased the effect of β_2-receptor activation in precontracted canine airways (103). The mechanism may be related to the opposing effects of M_2 and β_2 receptors on potassium ion flux across epithelial membranes and cellular membrane potentials. G_s proteins activated by β_2 receptors open a Ca^{2+}-dependent K^+ channel, leading to a flux of K^+ out of the cell (Fig. 6). The decreased intracellular K^+ concentration promotes smooth muscle relaxation. In contrast, M_2

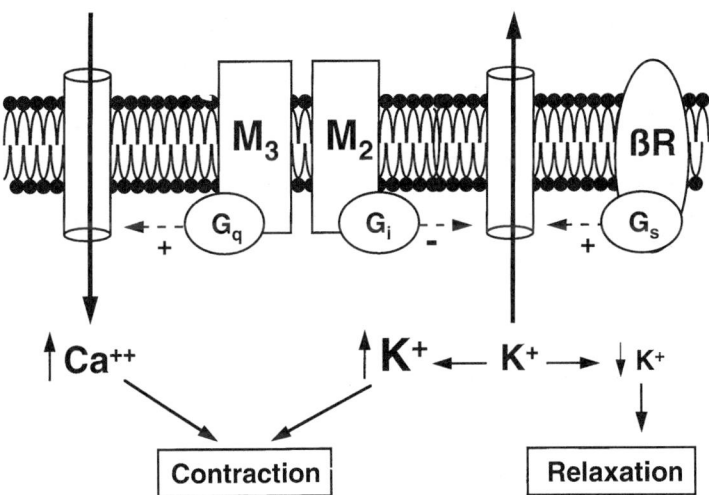

Figure 6 Hypothetical relationships between muscarinic and β_2-adrenergic receptors and ion channels in airways. M_3 receptors activate G_q proteins that activate Ca^{2+} influx. β_2-adrenergic receptors open, while M_2 receptors close; Ca^{2+}-dependent K^+ channels. These ionic fluxes regulate smooth muscle contraction and relaxation.

receptors activate G_i proteins that tend to close these Ca^{2+}-dependent K^+ channels, leading to intracellular hyperkalemia that promotes smooth muscle contraction. This effect may be compounded by the increase of intracellular calcium induced by M_3 receptors and their G_q proteins, leading to contraction. This hypothesis remains to be demonstrated in human airways, but may represent an additional mechanism of M_3 and M_2 receptor synergism to promote contraction.

M_2 receptor dysfunction on postganglionic neurons may account for the increased cholinergic bronchoconstrictor tone in airway inflammation. Inhalation of airway irritants and release of high levels of inflammatory mediators would provide a strong preganglionic signal. Loss of inhibitory M_2 autoreceptor function would reduce the "electric filtering" capacity of the ganglion cells and permit faster depolarization rates, increased postganglionic ACh release, and subsequent smooth muscle contraction. These changes could be manifest by the clinical finding of bronchial hyperresponsiveness after inhalation of methacholine, histamine, and hypertonic saline. This hypothesis is supported by the increased sensitivity of asthmatics to SO_2 and propanolol. SO_2 may stimulate mast cells and/or nociceptive sensory nerves and recruit parasympathetic reflexes to induce bronchoconstriction. Propranolol could block inhibitory β_2-adrenergic autoreceptors on ganglionic, but could also block the tonic bronchodilator tone of endogenous catecholamines. Asthmatics are less responsive to pilocarpine than normal subjects. Pilocarpine stimulates M_2 receptors and should reduce parasympathetic bronchoconstrictor tone. This activity is reduced in asthmatics. These findings suggest that decreases in inhibitory M_2 autoreceptor function in airway inflammation lead to increased cholinergic reflex-mediated bronchoconstriction (57,63,68).

In contrast to M_3 receptors, M_2 receptor expression is downregulated by nonselective muscarinic agonists and β_2-adrenergic agonists (104,105). Because of the inhibitory effects of M_2 agonists on adenylyl cyclase, these drugs may interfere with the relaxatory effects of β_2-agonists in vivo and in vitro (103,106).

Other factors may also modulate M_2 receptor expression during inflammation. TGF-β_1 induces transcriptional downregulation of m_2 receptor mRNA in a human embryonic lung fibroblast cell line (HEL 299) that expressed only M_2 receptors (107). In the same cells, the mixture of TNF-α and IL-1β inhibits the expression of M_2 receptors (108). Each cytokine had no effect on its own. Mast cell degranulation does not alter muscarinic receptor expression in human lung fragments in vitro (109), although these studies would not have been able to detect small changes in receptor subtype expression on ganglia in airways.

If M_2 receptor dysfunction is a component of the increased cholinergic tone in asthma and other inflammatory states, then changes in M_2 function should occur during allergen challenge. This has been examined in ovalbumin-sensitized guinea pigs that develop immediate (0- to 5-hour) and late (8- to 23-hour) phase bronchoconstriction after challenge. Bronchial hyperreactivity of methacholine and histamine and neutrophil and eosinophil infiltration develop (110). M_2 autoreceptor function was lost during the immediate allergic phase, but recovered after the late-phase response (111). The association among the severity of the immediate bronchoconstriction, inflammatory cell infiltration, and M_2 receptor dysfunction suggests that common mechanisms contribute to these effects. Polyanionic compounds such as heparin and poly-L-glutamate can prevent the M_2 dysfunction, possibly by binding to cationic proteins major basic protein (MBP) or eosinophil peroxidase (EPO) (112). In human heart membranes that contain M_2 receptors and in submandibular gland membranes that contain M_3 receptors, MBP (and, more weakly, EPO,) inhibits the binding the N-methyl-scopolamine to M_2, but not M_3, receptors. These effects were reversed by adding heparin. These data indicate that MBP and EPO are allosteric antagonists of M_2 receptors that may promote cholinergically mediated bronchoconstriction by inhibiting the capacity of M_2 to reduce postganglionic neuron depolarization (113).

XII. Summary

M_3 and M_2 receptors are the predominate muscarinic subtypes in the human respiratory tract. m_1 Receptor mRNA is present in unidentified alveolar cells, but not bronchi. m_2 mRNA is found in smooth muscle and ganglion cells. m_3 mRNA is found in bronchial epithelium, endothelium, glands, and smooth muscle. m_4 and m_5 mRNA are not detectable. M_3 receptor protein activation is the major tonically active stimulus for smooth muscle contraction and glandular exocytosis. M_3 antagonists may be beneficial, selective inhibitors of glandular secretion and vasodilation in human nasal mucosa and bronchoconstriction in human bronchi that may be free of side effects caused by actions on M_2 and other subtype receptors. M_2 receptors appear to be critical for the regulation of parasympathetic ganglion function since M_2 autoreceptor stimulation may reduce acetylcholine release. On smooth muscle, M_2 agonists may enhance cholinergically induced contraction by antagonizing cAMP formation and the relaxant effects of β_2-adrenergic agonists. These M_2 autoreceptor events may be at odds with each other, since ganglionic effects would promote bronchodilation and reduce cholinergically induced glandular secretion, while smooth muscle effects would promote bronchoconstriction.

The success of cholinergic antagonists in chronic asthma and chronic bronchitis can be rationalized by this distribution of receptors. In human airways, cholinergic bronchoconstriction is most important in the larger bronchi; anticholinergic agents are useful to dilate large airways. However, constriction of smaller bronchi predominates in asthma. Since cholinergic innervation and constrictor tone are less important in these smaller airways, anticholinergic drugs are less effective. β_2-Adrenergic agonists are more effective bronchodilators in small airways because they can actively induce smooth muscle relaxation. In contrast, COPD is characterized by irreversible airways obstruction with glandular hypersecretion. Anticholinergic drugs are effective at reducing cholinergically-mediated glandular secretion in proximal airways, while β_2-adrenergic agonists are less effective. However, because atropine, ipratropium bromide, and other currently available anticholinergic agents are nonselective, they block all muscarinic receptors, and so inhibit each of these cholinergically-mediated mechanisms. It is anticipated that pure M_3 antagonists without M_2 inhibitory activity would be more beneficial in asthma, chronic bronchitis, and other respiratory diseases, and that therapies directed at protecting M_2 inhibitory autoreceptors on bronchial ganglia would reduce cholinergic bronchial tone during eosinophilic inflammation.

Acknowledgments

Dr. Mullol was supported in part by Generalitat de Catalunya (CIRIT) and Fundació Catalana de Pneumologia (FUCAP). Dr. Baraniuk was supported by NIH RO1 AI 42403.

References

1. Barnes PJ. Modulation of neurotransmission in airways. Physiol Rev 1992; 72: 699.
2. Caulfield MP. Muscarinic receptors—characterization, coupling and function. Pharmacol Ther 1993; 58:319.
3. Eglen RM, Reddy H, Watson N, Challiss RAI. Muscarinic acetylcholine receptor subtypes in smooth muscle. TiPS 1994; 15:114.
4. Dey RD, Altemus JB, Rodd A, Mayer B, Said SI, Coburn RF. Neurochemical characterization of intrinsic neurons in ferret tracheal plexus. Am J Respir Cell Mol Biol 1996; 14:207–216.

5. Kummer W, Fischer A, Lang RE, Lin X, Koesling D, Mayer B, Olry R. Nitric oxide and guanylyl cyclases: correlation with neuropeptides. In: Kaliner MA, Barnes PJ, Kunkel GHH, Baraniuk JN, eds. Neuropeptides in Respiratory Medicine. New York: Marcel-Dekker, 1994: 641–652.
6. Barnes PJ, Baraniuk JN, Belvisi MG. Neuropeptides in the respiratory tract. Part 1. Am Rev Respir Dis 1991; 144:1187–1198.
7. Barnes PJ, Baraniuk JN, Belvisi MG. Neuropeptides in the respiratory tract. Part 2. Am Rev Respir Dis 1991; 144:1391–1399.
8. Springall DR, Polak JM, Howarth PH. Persistence of intrinsic neurones and possible phenotypic changes after extrinsic denervation of human respiratory tract by heart-lung transplantation. Am Rev Respir Dis 1990; 141:1538.
9. Lammers JW, Minette M, McCusker M, Barnes PJ. The role of pirenzepine-sensitive (M_1) muscarinic receptors in vagally mediated bronchoconstriction in humans. Am Rev Respir Dis 1989; 139:446–449.
10. Hokfelt T, Fuxe K, Pernow B. Coexistence of neuronal messengers: a new principle in chemical transmission. Prog Brain Res 1987; 68:1.
11. Lundberg JM, Angaard A, Fahrenkrug J. Complementary role of vasoactive intestinal peptide (VIP) and acetylcholine for cat submandibular gland blood flow and secretion. Acta Physiol Scand 1981; 113:329.
12. Uddman R, Sundler F. Innervation of the upper airways. Clin Chest Med 1986; 7:201.
13. Raphael GR, Baraniuk JN, Kaliner MA. How and why the nose runs. J Allergy Clin Immunol 1991; 87:457.
14. Baraniuk JN. Neural control of human nasal secretion. Pulm Pharmacol 1991; 4:20.
15. Richardson JB. Nerve supply to the lungs. Am Rev Respir Dis 1979; 119:785.
16. Partanen M, Laitinen A, Hervonen A, Toivanen M, Laitinen LA. Catecholine- and acetylcholinesterase-containing nerves in human lower respiratory tract. Histochemistry 1992; 76:175.
17. Laitinen LA, Laitinen A. Innervation or airway smooth muscle. Am Rev Respir Dis 1987; 136:S38.
18. Coles SJ, Said SI, Reid LM. Inhibition by vasoactive intestinal peptides of glycoconjugate and lysozyme secretion by human airways in vitro. Am Rev Respir Dis 1981; 124:531.
19. Marom Z, Goswami SK. Respiratory mucus hypersecretion (bronchorrea): a case discussion—possible mechanism(s) and treatment. J Allergy Clin Immunol 1991; 87:1050.
20. Ollerenshaw S, Jarvis D, Woolcock A, Sullivan C, Scheibner T. Absence of immunoreactive vasoactive intestinal peptide in tissue from the lungs of patients with asthma. N Engl J Med 1989; 320:1244.
21. Heinz-Erian P, Dev RD, Said SI. Deficient vasoactive intestinal peptide innervation in sweat glands of cystic fibrosis patients. Science 1985; 229:1407.
22. Kurian SS, Blank MA, Sheppard MN. Vasoactive intestinal polypeptide (VIP) in vasomotor rhinitis. Clin Biochem 1983; 11:425.

23. Stjarne P, Lacroix JS, Anggard A, Lundberg JM. Compartment analysis of vascular effects of neuropeptides and capsaicin in the pig nasal mucosa. Acta Physiol Scand 1991; 141:335.
24. Barnes PJ, Nadel JA, Roberts JM, Basbaum CB: Muscarinic receptors in lung and trachea: autradiographic localization using [^{3}H]quinuclidinyl benzilate. Eur J Pharmacol 1983; 86:103.
25. Mak JCW, Barnes PJ. Muscarinic receptor subtypes in human and guinea pig lung. Eur J Pharmacol 1989; 164:223.
26. Mak JCW, Barnes PJ. Autoradiographic visualization of muscarinic receptor subtypes in human and guinea pig lung. Am Rev Respir Dis 1990; 141:1559.
27. Van Koppen CJ, Rodrigues de Miranda JF, Beld AJ, Hermanussen MW, Lammers J-WJ, Van Ginneken CAM. Characterization of the muscarinic receptor in human tracheal smooth muscle. Arch Pharmacol 1985; 331:247.
28. Van Koppen CJ, Blankesteijn WM, Klassen ABM, Rodrigues de Miranda JF, Beld AJ, Van Ginneken CAM. Autoradiographic visualization of muscarinic receptors in human bronchi. J Pharmacol Exp Ther 1988; 244:760.
29. Okayama M, Baraniuk JN, Merida M, Kaliner MA. Autoradiographic localization of muscarinic receptor subtypes in human nasal mucosa. J Allergy Clin Immunol 1992; 89:1144.
30. Barnes PJ. Muscarinic receptor subtypes in airways. Life Sci 1993; 52:521–527.
31. Mak JCW, Baraniuk JN, Barnes PJ. Localization of muscarinic receptor subtype messenger RNA's in human lung. Am J Respir Cell Mol Biol 1992; 7:344.
32. Zaagsma J, Roffel AF, Meurs H. Muscarinic control of airway function. Life Sci 1997; 60:1061–1068.
33. Haxhiu-Poskurica B, Ernsberger P, Haxhiu MA, Miller MJ, Cattarossi L, Martin RJ. Development of cholinergic innervation and muscarinic receptor subtypes in piglet trachea. Am J Physiol 1993; 264:L606.
34. Baraniuk JN, Kaliner MA, Barnes PJ. Muscarinic m3 receptor mRNA in situ hybridization in human nasal mucosa. Am J Rhinol 1992; 6:145.
35. Dale HH. The action of certain esters and ethers of choline, and their relation to muscarine. J Pharmacol Exp Ther 1914; 6:147–190.
36. Buckley NJ, Bonner TI, Buckley CM, Brann MR. Antagonist binding properties of five cloned muscarinic receptors expressed in CHO-K1 cells. Mol Pharmacol 1989; 35:469.
37. Dorje F, Wess J, Lambrecht G, Tacke R, Mutschler E, Brann MR. Antagonist binding profiles of five cloned human muscarinic receptor subtypes. J Pharmacol Exp Ther 1991; 256:727.
38. Eglen RM, Hegde SS, Watson N. Muscarinic receptor subtypes and smooth muscle function. Pharmacol Rev 1996; 48:531–565.
39. Fraser CM, Lee NH. Molecular characterization of autonomic and neuropeptide receptors. In: Kaliner MA, Barnes PJ, Kunkel GHH, Baraniuk JN, eds. Neuropeptides in Respiratory Medicine. New York: Marcel-Dekker 1994:225–250.

40. Hosey MM. Diversity of structure, signalling and regulation within the family of muscarinic cholinergic receptors. FASEB J 1992; 6:845–852.
41. Kurtenbach E, Curtis CAM, Pedder EK. Muscarinic acetylcholine receptors. Peptide sequencing isentifies residues involved in antagonist binding and disulfide bond formation. J Biol Chem 1990; 265:13702.
42. Fraser CM, Wang C-D, Robinson DA. Site-directed mutagenesis of m_1 muscarinic receptors: conserved aspartic acids play important roles in receptor function. Mol Pharmacol 1989; 36:840.
43. Wess J, Nanavati S, Vogel Z. Functional role of proline and tryptophan residues highly conserved among G protein-coupled receptors studied by mutational analysis of the m_3 muscarinic receptor EMBO J 1992; 12:331.
44. Norvald G, Hacksell U. Binding site modelling of the muscarinic m_1 receptor: a combination of homology-based and indirect approaches. J Med Chem 1993; 36:967.
45. Hibert MF, Trumpp-Kallmeyer S, Bruinvels A, Hoflack J. Three-dimensional models of neurotransmitter G-binding protein-coupled receptors. Mol Pharm 1991; 40:8.
46. Duerson K, Carroll R, Clapham D. Alpha-helical distorting substitution disrupt coupling between m_3 and muscarinic receptor and G proteins. FEBS Lett 1993; 324:103.
47. Yang CM, Chow S-P, Sung T-C. Muscarinic receptor subtypes coupled to generation of different second messengers in isolated tracheal smooth muscle cells. Br J Pharmacol 1991; 104:613.
48. Felder CC. Muscarinic acetylcholine receptor signal transduction through multiple effectors. FASEB J 1995; 9:619–625.
49. Beck KC, Vettermann J, Flavahan NA, Rehder K. Muscarinic M_1 receptors mediate the increase in pulmonary resistance during vagus nerve stimulation in dogs. Am Rev Respir Dis 1987; 137:1135.
50. Bloom JW, Yamamura HI, Baumgartner C, Halonen M. A muscarinic receptor with high affinity for pirenzepine mediates vagally induced bronchoconstriction. Eur J Pharmacol 1987; 133:21.
51. Lammers J-WJ, Minette P, MuCusker M, Barnes PJ. The role of pirenzepine-sensitive (M_1) muscarinic receptors in vagally mediated bronchoconstriction in humans. Am Rev Respir Dis 1989; 139:446.
52. Ishihara H, Shimura S, Satoh M, et al. Muscarinic receptor subtypes in feline tracheal submucosal gland secretion. Am J Physiol 1992; 262 (Lung Cell Mol Physiol 6):L223–L228.
53. Mullol J, Baraniuk JN, Logun C, et al. M_1 and M_3 muscarinic antagonists inhibit human nasal glandular secretion in vitro. J Appl Physiol 1992; 73:2069–2073.
54. Bloom JW, Halonen M, Yamamura HI. Characterization of muscarinic cholinergic receptor subtypes in human peripheral lung. J Pharmacol Exp Ther 1988; 244:625.
55. Maeda A, Kubo T, Mishina M, Numa S. Tissue distribution if mRNAa encoding mescarinic acetylcholine receptor subtypes. FEBS Lett 1988; 239:339.

56. Griffin MT, Ehlert FJ. Specific inhibition of isoproterenol cyclic AMP accumulation by M_2 muscarinic receptors in rat intestinal smooth muscle. J Pharm Exp Ther 1992; 263:221.
57. Minette PA, Barnes PJ. Prejunctional inhibitory muscarinic receptors on cholinergic nerves in human and guinea pig airways. J Appl Physiol 1988; 64: 2532.
58. Fryer AD, Jacoby DB. Effect of inflammatory cell mediators on M_2 muscarinic receptors in the lungs. Life Sci 1993; 52:529–536.
59. Kilbinger H, Schoreider R, Siefken H, Wolf D, D'Agostino G. Characterization of prejunctional muscarinic autoreceptors in the guinea-pig trachea. Br J Pharmacol 1991; 103:1757.
60. Fryer AD, Maclagan J. Muscarinic inhibitory receptors in pulmonary parasympathetic nerves in the guinea pig. Br J Pharmacol 1984; 83:973.
61. Patel HJ, Barnes PJ, Takehashi T, Tadjkarimi S, Yacoub MH, Belvisi MG. Evidence for prejunctional muscarinic autoreceptors in human and guinea pig trachea. Am J Respir Crit Care Med 1995; 152:872–878.
62. Fryer AD, Costello RW, Yost BY, et al. Antibody to VLA-4, but not to L-selectin, protects neuronal M_2 muscarinic receptors in antigen challenged guinea pig airways. J Clin Invest 1997; 99:2036–2044.
63. Minette PAH, Lanners J, Dixon CMS, McCuster MT, Barnes PJ. A muscarinic agonist inhibits reflex bronchoconstriction in normal but not in asthmatic subjects. J Appl Physiol 1989; 67:2461.
64. Racke K, Hey C, Wessler I. Endogenous noradrenaline release from guinea pig isolated trachea is inhibited by activation of M_2 receptors. Br J Pharmacol 1992; 107:3.
65. Fryer AD, Jacoby DB. Parainfluenza virus infection damages inhibitory M_2 muscarinic receptors on pulmonary parasympathetic nerves in the guinea-pig. Br J Pharmacol 1991; 102:267.
66. Haddad E-B, Gies JP. Neuraminidase reduces the super-high-affinity [^{3}H]oxotremorine-M binding sites in guinea pig. Eur J Pharmacol 1992; 211:L327.
67. Fryer AD, Wills-Karp M. Dysfunction of M_2 receptors in pulmonary parasympathetic nerves after allergen challenge in guinea pigs. J Appl Physiol 1991; 71:2255–2261.
68. Ayala LE, Ahmed T. Is there loss of a protective muscarinic receptor in asthma? Chest 1989; 96:1285–1291.
69. Costello RW, Schofield BH, Kephart GM, Gleich GJ, Jacoby DB, Fryer AD. Localization of eosinophils to airway nerves, and effect on neuronal M_2 muscarinic receptor function. Am J Physiol 1997; 273:L93–103.
70. Elbon CL, Jacoby DB, Fryer AD. Pretreatment with an antibody to interleukin-5 prevents loss of pulmonary M_2 muscarinic receptor function in antigen challenged guinea pigs. Am J Respir Cell Mol Biol 1995; 12:320–328.
71. Evans CM, Jacoby DB, Gleich GJ, Fryer AD, Costello RW. Antibody to eosinophil major basic protein protects M_2 receptor function in antigen challenged guinea pigs in vivo. J Clin Invest 1997; 100:2254–2262.

72. Jacoby DB, Gleich GJ, Fryer AD. Human eosinophil major basic protein is and endogenous, allosteric antagonist at the inhibitory muscarinic M^2 receptor. Am Rev Respir Dis 1992; 145:A436.
73. Diamant Z, Timmers MC, Van der Veen H, Page CP, Van der Meer FJ, Sterk PJ. Effect of inhaled heparin on allergen-induced early and late asthmatic responses in patients with atopic asthma. Am J Respir Crit Care Med 1996; 153: 1790–1795.
74. Fryer AD, Jacoby DB. Function of pulmonary M_2 muscarinic receptors in antigen challenged guinea pigs is restored by heparin and poly-L-glutamate. J Clin Invest 1992; 90:2292–2298.
75. Schultheis A, Bassett DJP, Fryer AD. Ozone induced airway hyperresponsiveness is due to temporary loss of neuronal M_2 muscarinic receptor function. Am Rev Respir Dis 1992; 145:A615.
76. Fryer A, Okanlami O. Neuronal M_2 muscarinic receptor function in guinea pig lungs in inhibited by indomethacin. Am Rev Respir Dis 1993; 147:500.
77. Stechschulte DJ. Leukotrienes in asthma and allergic rhinitis. N Engl J Med 1990; 323:1769.
78. Grandordy BM, Cuss FM, Sampson AS, Palmer JB, Barnes PJ. Phosphatidylinositol response to cholinergic agonists in airway smooth muscle: relationship to contaction and muscarinic receptor occupancy. J Pharmacol Exp Ther 1986; 238:273.
79. Chilvers ER, Batty IH, Barnes PJ, Nahorski SR. Formation of inositol polyphosphates in airway smooth muscle after muscarinic receptor stimulation. J Pharmacol Exp Ther 1990; 252:786.
80. Roux F, Mavoungov E, Naline E, et al. Role of 1,2-sn diacylglycerol in airway smooth muscle stimulated by carbachol. Am J Respir Crit Care Med 1995; 151: 1745–1751.
81. Williams CL, Hayes VY, Hummmel AM, Tarara JE, Halsey TJ. Regulation of E-cadherin-mediated adhesion by muscarinic acetylcholine receptors in small cell carcinoma. J Cell Biol 1993; 121:643–654.
82. McCormack DG, Mak JC, Minette P, Barnes PJ. Muscarinic receptor subtypes mediating vasodilation in the pulmonary artery. Eur J Pharmacol 1993; 158: 293.
83. Tokuyama K, Kuo H-P, Rohode JAL, Barnes PJ, Rogers DF. Neural control of goblet cell secretion in guinea pig airways. Am J Physiol (Lung Cell Mol Physiol) 1990; 259:L108.
84. Yu DYC, Galant SP, Gold WM. Inhibition of antigen-induced bronchoconstriction by atropine in asthmatic patients. J Appl Physiol 1972; 32:823.
85. Alabaster VA. Discovery and development of selective M_3 antagonists for clinical use. Life Sci 1997; 60:1053–1060.
86. Mak JCW, Haddad EB, Buckley NJ, Barnes PJ. Visualization of muscarinic m4 mRNA and M_4 receptor subtype in rabbit lung. Life Sci 1993; 53: 1501.
87. Kilbinger H, Von Barbeleben RS, Siefken H. Is the presynaptic muscarinic

autoreceptor in the guinea-pig trachea an M_2 receptor? (abstract). Life Sci 1993; 52:577.
88. Van Megen YJB, Klaassen ABM, Rodrigues de Miranda JF, Van Ginneken CAM, Wentges BTR. Alterations of muscarinic acetylcholine receptors in the nasal mucosa of allergic patients in comparison with nonallergic individuals. J Allergy Clin Immunol 1991; 87:521.
89. Baraniuk JN, Kaliner MA, Barnes PJ. Muscarinic m3 receptor mRNA in situ hybridization in human nasal mucosa. Am J Rhinol 1992; 6:145.
90. Yang B, McCaffrey TV. The roles of muscarinic receptor subtypes in modulation of nasal ciliary action. Rhinology 1996; 34:136–139.
91. Mygind N, Borum P. Anticholinergic treatment of watery rhinorrhea. Am J Rhinol 1990; 4:1.
92. Druce HM, Wright RH, Kossoff D, Kaliner MA. Cholinergic nasal hyperreactivity in atopic subjects. J Allergy Clin Immunol 1985; 76:445.
93. Devillier P, Dessanges JF, Rakatosihanaka J, Ghaem A, Boushey HA, Lockhart A. Nasal response to substance P and methacholine in subjects with and without allergic rhinitis. Eur Respir J 1988; 1:356.
94. Stjarne P, Lundblad L, Lundberg JM, Anggard A. Capsaicin and nicotine sensitive afferent neurones and nasal secretion in healthy human volunteers and in patients with vasomotor rhinitis. Br J Pharmacol 1989; 96:693.
95. Molfino NA, Slutsky AS, Julia-Serda G, et al. Assessment of airway tone in asthma. Comparison between double lung transplant patients and healthy subjects. Am Rev Respir Dis 1993; 148:1238–1243.
96. Robertson DN, Rhoden KJ, Grandordy B, Page CP, Barnes PJ. The effect of platelet activating factor on histamine and muscarinic receptor function in guinea pig airways. Am Rev Respir Dis 1988; 137:1317.
97. Roberts JA, Raeburn D, Rodger IW, Thomson NC. Comparison of in vivo airway responsiveness and in vitro smooth muscle sensitivity to methacholine. Thorax 1984; 39:837.
98. Van Koppen CJ, Rodrigues de Miranda JF, Beld AJ, et al. Muscarinic receptor sensitivity in airway smooth muscle of patients with obstructive airway disease. Arch Int Pharmacodyn Ther 1988; 295:238.
99. Van Koppen CJ, Lammers J-WJ, Rodrigues de Miranda JF, et al. Muscarinic receptor binding in central airway musculature in chronic airflow limitation. Pulm Pharmacol 1988; 2:131.
100. Whicker SD, Armour CL, Black JL. Responsiveness of bronchial smooth muscle from asthmatic patients to relaxant and contractile agonists. Pulm Pharmacol 1988; 1:25.
101. Haddad EB, Mak JCW, Belvisi MG, Nishikawa M, Rousell J, Barnes PJ. Muscarinic and beta-adrenergic receptor expression in peripheral lung from normal and asthmatic patients. Am J Physiol (Lung) 1996; 270:L947–L953.
102. Watson N, Magnussen H, Rabe KF. Antagonism of beta-adrenoreceptor mediated relaxations of human bronchial smooth muscle by carbachol. Eur J Pharmacol 1995; 275:307–310.

103. Fernandes LB, Fryer AD, Hirschman CA. M_2 muscarinic receptors inhibit isoproterenol-induced relaxation of canine smooth muscle. J Pharmacol Exp Ther 1992; 262:119–126.
104. Haddad EB, Roussel J, Mak JCW, Barnes PJ. Long-term carbachol treatment induced down-regulation of muscarinic M_2 receptors but not m2 receptor mRNA in a human lung cell line. Br J Pharmacol 1995; 116:2027–2032.
105. Roussel J, Haddad EB, Mak JCW, Webb BL, Giembycz MA, Barnes PJ. Beta-adrenoceptor mediated down-regulation of M_2 muscarinic receptors: role of cyclic adenosine 5′ monophosphate-dependent protein kinase. J Mol Pharmacol 1996; 49:629–635.
106. Yang CM, Chou SP, Sung TC. Muscarinic receptor subtypes coupled to generation of different second messengers in isolated tracheal smooth muscle cells. Br J Pharmacol 1991; 104:613–618.
107. Haddad EB, Roussel J, Mak JCW, Barnes PJ. Transforming growth factor beta 1 induces transcriptional downregulation of m2 muscarinic receptor gene expression. Mol Pharmacol 1996; 49:781–787.
108. Haddad EB, Rousell J, Barnes PJ. Synergy between tumor necrosis factor alpha and interleukin 1-beta in inducing transcriptional downregulation of muscarinic m2 receptor gene expression. J Biol Chem 1996; 271:32586–32596.
109. Casale TB. Acute effects of in vitro mast cell degranulation on human lung muscarinic receptors. Am Rev Respir Dis 1993; 147:940.
110. Santing RE, Olymulder CG, Zaagsma J, Meurs H. Relationships among allergen induced early and late phase airway obstruction, bronchial hyperreactivity, and inflammation in conscious, unrestrained guinea pigs. J Allergy Clin Immunol 1994; 93:1021–1030.
111. Ten Berge RE, Santing RE, Hamstra JJ, Roffel AF, Zaagsma J. Dysfunction of muscarinic M_2 receptors after the early allergic reaction: possible contribution to bronchial hyperresponsiveness in allergic guinea pigs. Br J Pharmacol 1995; 114:881–887.
112. Fryer AD, Jacoby DB. Function of pulmonary M_2 muscarinic recpeots in antigen-challenged guinae pigs is restored by heparin and poly-L-glutamate. J Clin Invest 1992; 90:2292–2298.
113. Jacoby DB, Gleich GJ, Fryer AD. Human eosinophil major basic protein is an endogeneous allosteric antagonist at the inhibitory muscarinic M_2 receptor. J Clin Invest 1993; 91:1314–1318.

2

Airway Muscarinic Receptors

PETER J. BARNES

National Heart and Lung Institute
Imperial College
London, England

I. Introduction

Cholinergic antagonists are now widely used in the treatment of obstructive airways diseases and may be the bronchodilators of choice in the treatment of COPD, where cholinergic tone is the only reversible component. The recognition that there are multiple subtypes of muscarinic receptor in lung has raised important questions about their role in regulation of airway function, and creates the prospect of more selective therapy in the future (1). Five distinct human muscarinic receptor genes have so far been identified (2), and four subtypes of muscarinic receptor (M_1 to M_4) have now been recognized in lung both pharmacologically and using specific cDNA probes (3–7) (Fig. 1). These subtypes of muscarinic receptor subserve different physiological roles in the airways, but their clinical relevance in the treatment of airway disease is not yet certain.

The vagus nerve releases acetylcholine which activates muscarinic receptors on smooth muscle and submucosal gland cells, which results in bron-

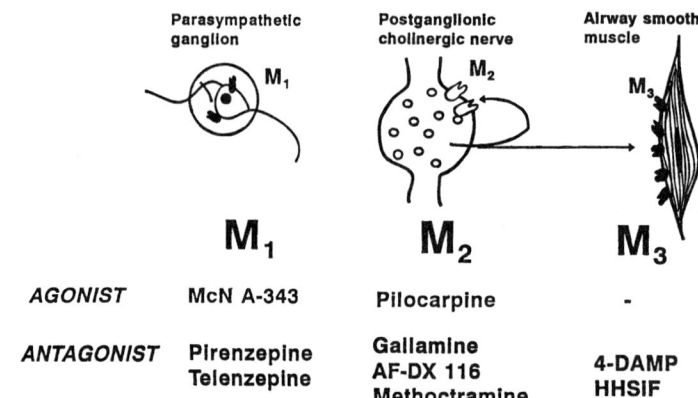

Figure 1 Muscarinic receptor subtypes.

choconstriction and mucus secretion, respectively (8). Muscarinic receptors regulate the secretion of mucus from both submucosal glands and airway epithelial goblet cells (9). Autoradiographic mapping studies using [^{3}H]quinuclidinyl benzylate indicate that muscarinic receptors are predominantly localized to airway smooth muscle, vascular endothelium, submucosal gland cells, and neuronal structures (10–12), although in some species, including humans, there is also localization to alveolar walls.

Binding studies with lung homogenates indicate that there is a high proportion of pirenzepine-sensitive binding sites, presumed to be M_1 receptors in several species, including humans and rabbits (13–15). In human lung membrane high-affinity pirenzepine-sensitive sites make up approximately 70% of total binding, which is confirmed by studies using [^{3}H]pirenzepine as a radioligand (15). Autoradiographic mapping studies indicate that these receptors are localized to the alveolar walls (11). Other species, such as guinea pig and ferret, do not appear to have these parenchymal muscarinic receptors (10,11), but their significance is far from clear as there is no evidence for cholinergic innervation of the lung periphery. Recently it has been found that in some species epithelial cells have the capacity to secrete acetylcholine, raising the possibility that muscarinic receptors in the airways may be activated by acetylcholine derived from nonneuronal sources (16).

Three distinct subtypes of receptor have now been recognized pharmacologically. M_1 receptors are pirenzepine-sensitive and are usually localized to neuronal structures. M_2 receptors are present in atrium and mediate the heart-rate slowing with cholinergic stimulation. M_2 receptors are selectively blocked by AF-DX 116, methoctramine, or gallamine, and are clearly different from muscarinic receptors on smooth muscle (M_3 receptors), which are sensitive to 4-diphenylocetoxy-N-methyl-piperidine methiodide (4-DAMP) and hexahydrosiladifenidol. All three muscarinic receptor subtypes have now been described in airways (1,5), but their possible relevance to airway disease and therapy is not yet certain.

II. M_1 Receptors

The discovery that the muscarinic antagonist pirenzepine was able to discriminate between high- and low-affinity muscarinic receptor binding sites (17) supported previous suggestions that subtypes of muscarinic receptor might exist. Receptors with a high affinity for pirenzepine, which are designated M_1 receptors, are found in cerebral cortex and autonomic ganglia, in contrast to lower-affinity receptors which predominate in heart and smooth muscle (which were therefore called M_2 receptors). Pirenzepine is used clinically to reduce gastric acid secretion and, while it was previously believed to act directly on acid-secreting cells, it is now clear that it acts predominantly on ganglia in the stomach to inhibit neurally mediated gastric secretion (18). Since the innervation of the airways is derived embryologically from that of the gut, it seemed likely that excitatory M_1 receptors might also exist in airway ganglia. There appear to be considerable species differences in the location of muscarinic receptors in pulmonary nerves, however. In vitro, pirenzepine has a low affinity for acetylcholine-induced contraction of rabbit airways (19) and for binding of the nonselective antagonist [^{3}H]quinuclidinyl benzilate (QNB) to bovine airways (20,21), suggesting that M_1 receptors are not present in airway smooth muscle. Similarly, pirenzepine is only weakly effective in inhibiting cholinergic agonist-stimulated phosphoinositide turnover in bovine airway smooth muscle (20,21).

Pirenzepine is a bronchodilator when given intravenously to human subjects (22), although at the dose used it might be acting nonselectively and blocking smooth muscle muscarinic receptors. Lower doses of intravenous pirenzepine, while having no effect on FEV_1, increases expired flow at low lung volumes, suggesting an effect on more peripheral airways (23). This might be consistent with the existence of M_1 receptors in peripheral but not central human airways. Another M_1-selective antagonist telenzepine gave no significant clinical benefits in patients with COPD, however (24).

M_1 receptors may also be present in human airway cholinergic nerves. The effects of inhaled pirenzepine and ipratropium bromide were studied on cholinergic reflex bronchoconstriction triggered by the inhalation of the irritant gas sulfur dioxide in allergic volunteers (25). A dose of inhaled pirenzepine was found that did not inhibit bronchoconstriction due to an inhaled cholinergic agonist (methacholine), whereas ipratropium bromide was able to block the bronchoconstrictor effect. The same dose of pirenzepine, however, was as effective as ipratropium bromide in blocking cholinergic reflex bronchoconstriction, and, since it could not be acting directly on airway smooth muscle receptors, it might be acting on some peripheral part of the cholinergic pathway, which is most likely to be parasympathetic ganglia in the airways. In support of this possibility, pirenzepine has been shown to depress cholinergic ganglionic neurotransmission in rabbit bronchi *in vitro* (26).

The physiological role of the M_1 receptors in ganglia is still not certain. Classically, ganglionic transmission is via nicotinic cholinergic receptors which are blocked by hexamethonium. It is possible that excitatory M_1 receptors are facilitatory to nicotinic receptors and may be involved in "setting" the efficacy of ganglionic transmission (Fig. 2). Activation of these receptors probably closes K^+ channels, resulting in a slow depolarization of the ganglion cell (27). Perhaps they might be involved in the chronic regulation of cholinergic tone, whereas nicotinic receptors are more important in rapid signaling, such as occurs during reflex activation of the cholinergic pathway. If so, then M_1 antagonists, such as pirenzepine and telenzepine, might have a useful therapeutic role in asthma and COPD, since they may reduce vagal tone. Since increased vagal tone may play a crucial role in nocturnal exacerbations of asthma, then pirenzepine might prove to be efficacious in preventing nocturnal wheeze.

The results of binding studies in lung are unexpected. Binding of [^{3}H]QNB to both rabbit and human peripheral lung membranes is displaced by pirenzepine with a shallow inhibitory curve, suggesting the presence of high- and low-affinity sites (13–15). The high-affinity binding site has the characteristic expected of an M_1 receptor, and this is confirmed by the use of [^{3}H]pirenzepine to label the receptors (15). M_1 receptors make up more than half of the binding sites in lung of both species, which cannot be accounted for by receptors on airway ganglia or nerves, which would make up only a small fraction of the membranes. Autoradiographic mapping studies suggest that M_1 receptors in human airways are present on submucosal glands and are also seen over alveolar walls (11). These autoradiographic studies have recently been supported by *in situ* hybridization studies using cDNA and oligonucleotide probes, which hybridize to the specific messenger RNA encoded by the genes for the different muscarinic receptor subtypes (6). In human lung M_1-receptor mRNA is localized to submucosal glands and to alveolar walls,

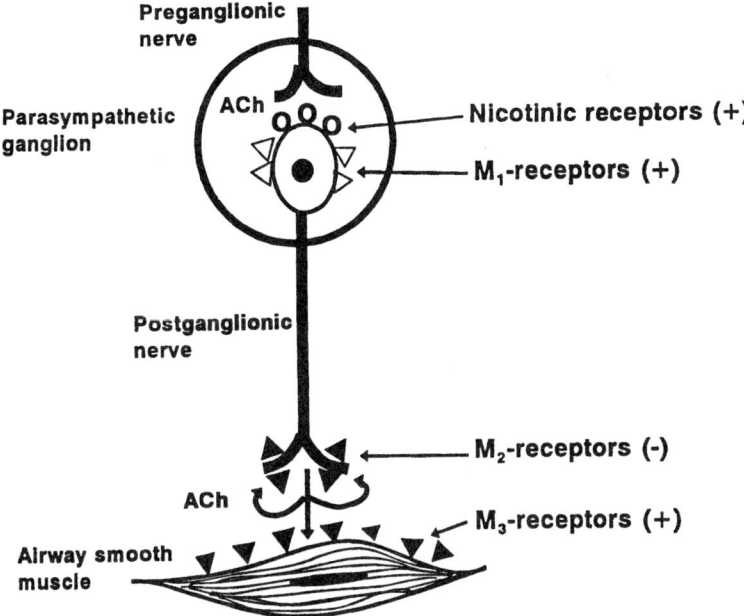

Figure 2 Muscarinic receptor subtypes in airways. Ganglionic neurotransmission is mediated via nicotinic receptors (ion channels), but M_1 receptors may facilitate this transmission. M_2 receptors on postganglionic cholinergic nerve terminals inhibit the release of acetylcholine (ACh), thus reducing the stimulation of postjunctional M_3 receptors which constrict airway smooth muscle.

whereas in rabbit lung the muscarinic receptors localized to the peripheral lung appear to belong to the M_4-receptor subtype (28).

III. M_2 Receptors

Binding studies of airway smooth muscle indicate a preponderance of M_2 receptors, which inhibit adenylyl cyclase (29,30) (Fig. 3). Recent studies indicate that these M_2 receptors may play a role in functional antagonism and counteract the bronchodilator action of β-agonists in some species (31,32), but this has not been seen in guinea pig or human airway smooth muscle (33,34). The functional role of M_2 receptors in these species is therefore uncer-

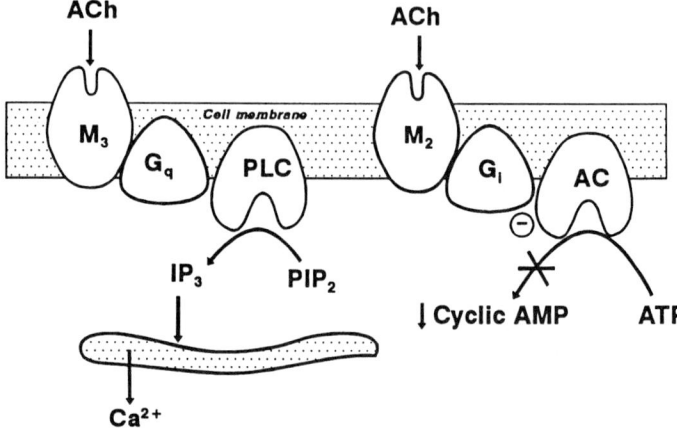

Figure 3 In airway smooth muscle M_2 and M_3 receptors are present. M_3 receptors are coupled via a G-protein (G_q) to phospholipase C (PLC), resulting in formation of inositol(1,4,5)trisphosphate (IP_3) and calcium ion (Ca^{2+}) release. M_2 receptors are negatively coupled via G_i to adenylyl cyclase (AC), resulting in a fall in intracellular cyclic AMP.

tain, but it is possible that these receptors may regulate some other function, such as proliferative responses.

A. Muscarinic Autoreceptors

Muscarinic autoreceptors that inhibit the release of acetylcholine from cholinergic nerves have been described in gut and airways (35). These receptors are inhibited by gallamine and are therefore classified as M_2 receptors, thus differing from the muscarinic receptor subtypes on airway smooth muscle which are classified as M_3 receptors. These muscarinic receptors appear to be located prejunctionally on postganglionic parasympathetic nerves (36) and have a powerful inhibitory influence on acetylcholine release. M_2 receptors are also expressed on cultured parasympathetic nerves (37). Muscarinic autoreceptors have been demonstrated in guinea pig (38–40), cat (41), rat (42), dog (43), and human (39) airways. Measurement of acetylcholine release in human airways has confirmed that these inhibitory autoreceptors are of the M_2-receptor subtype (44). In normal human subjects pilocarpine, which selectively stimulates prejunctional M_1 receptors, has an inhibitory effect on cholinergic reflex bronchoconstriction induced by SO_2, suggesting that these inhibitory receptors are present *in vivo* and presumably serve to limit cholinergic bronchoconstriction (45). Other evidence now also supports this observation (46,47). In asthmatic patients pilocarpine has no such inhibitory action, indicating that there might be some dysfunction of the autoreceptor, which would result in exaggerated cholinergic reflex bronchoconstriction (45,48).

A functional defect in muscarinic autoreceptors may also explain why β-adrenergic blockers produce such marked bronchoconstriction in asthmatic patients, since any increase in cholinergic tone due to blockade of inhibitory β-receptors on cholinergic nerves would normally be switched off by M_2 receptors in the nerves, and a lack of such receptors may lead to increased acetylcholine release, resulting in exaggerated bronchoconstriction (49) (Fig. 4). Support for this idea is provided by the protective effect of oxitropium bromide against propranolol-induced bronchoconstriction in asthmatic patients (50).

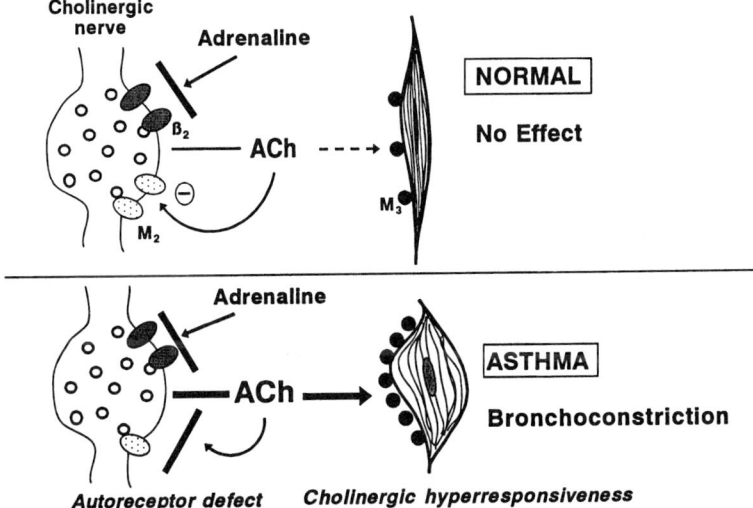

Figure 4 A possible mechanism of β-blocker-induced bronchoconstriction. β-blockers may inhibit the modulatory effect of circulating adrenaline on $β_2$-receptors of cholinergic nerves, thus increasing ACh release. In normal subjects this may act at M_2 autoreceptors to inhibit further ACh release, so no effect on airway smooth muscle is seen. In asthmatic patients, if there is a defect in M_2 receptors the increased ACh cannot switch itself off. Released ACh also has a greater effect on airway smooth muscle because of nonspecific airway hyperresponsiveness in asthma.

B. Mechanisms of M_2-Receptor Dysfunction

The mechanism by which M_2 autoreceptors on cholinergic nerves may become dysfunctional is not certain. It is possible that chronic inflammation in airways may lead to downregulation of M_2 receptors, which may have an important functional effect if the density of prejunctional muscarinic receptors is relatively low. Experimental studies have demonstrated that influenza virus may inactivate M_2 rather than M_3 receptors (51,52). This may be related to the action of viral neuraminidase on sialic acid residues of M_2 receptors (53). This provides a possible explanation for increased airway reactivity after influenza infections and the efficacy of anticholinergic bronchodilators during acute exacerbations of asthma, which are mainly virus-induced. Allergen challenge also results in M_2-receptor dysfunction (54,55), and this is blocked by an antibody to interleukin-5, suggesting that eosinophils are involved (56). Indeed, eosinophils appear to be particularly associated with cholinergic nerves in the airways of allergen-challenged guinea pigs and in patients with fatal asthma

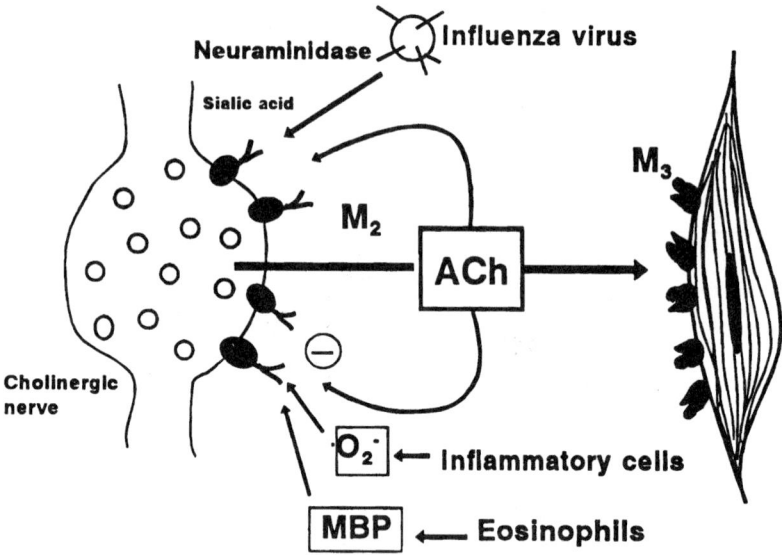

Figure 5 Muscarinic autoreceptors in disease. There may be a defect in M_2-receptor function in asthma, possibly due to effects of neuraminidase released in viral infection, or the effects of major basic protein (MBP) or superoxide anions (O_2^-) released by eosinophils. This would lead to increased release of ACh and therefore enhanced cholinergic neural bronchoconstriction.

(57). An antibody to the adhesion molecule VLA-4 blocks eosinophil recruitment after allergen exposure and also prevents M_2-receptor dysfunction (58). Eosinophil major basic protein (MBP) appears to interact with M_2 (but not M_3) receptors to result in impaired function of prejunctional receptors, and increased ACh release when cholinergic reflexes are activated (59) (Fig. 5). An antibody to MBP also blocks the effect of allergen on M_2 receptors (60). Ozone also impairs M_2-receptor function, and this is blocked by cyclophosphamide, indicating that inflammatory cell influx, presumably with neutrophils, is involved (61). Recent studies have suggested that several inflammatory mediators result in reduced transcription of the M_2-receptor gene (62). This mechanism may contribute to cholinergic bronchoconstriction in acute exacerbations of asthma.

IV. M_3 Receptors

Muscarinic receptors on airway smooth muscle are sensitive to 4-DAMP and hexahydrosiladifenidol and are therefore classified as M_3 receptors (30). Binding studies in guinea pig and human lung membranes indicate the presence of M_3 receptors (15). Autoradiographic studies have demonstrated M_3 receptors in airway smooth muscle of large and small human airways (11), and this has been confirmed by *in situ* hybridization studies with M_3-selective cDNA probes (6). In the airways, smooth muscle muscarinic receptor activation results in rapid phosphoinositide hydrolysis (20,63,64) and the formation of inositol-(1,4,5)-trisphosphate (65), which releases calcium ions from intracellular stores.

M_3 receptors are also localized to submucosal glands in human airways, which appear to have a mixed population of M_1 and M_3 receptors in a proportion of 1:2 (11,66). M_3-selective antagonists potently inhibit mucus glycoprotein secretion form human airways *in vitro*, suggesting that M_3 receptors predominate (67). M_3 receptors are only weakly expressed on airway epithelial cells (11), in contrast to the strong *in situ* hybridization signal with an m_3 receptor cDNA probe (6), indicating that there may be a very rapid turnover of receptors. A similar epithelial expression of m_3-receptor mRNA is found in human nasal biopsies (68). M_3 receptors are also localized to endothelial cells of the bronchial circulation and presumably mediate the vasodilator response to cholinergic stimulation of the proximal airways (69). The vasodilator response to acetylcholine in pulmonary vessels is mediated via an M_3 receptor on endothelial cells (70).

The expression of M_2 and M_3 receptors in canine airway smooth muscle is reduced by the glucocorticoid dexamethasone, suggesting that corticosteroid may reduce cholinergic responsiveness (71).

V. M_4 and M_5 Receptors

In rabbit lung there is evidence from binding studies for the existence of an M_4 receptor, and this has been confirmed by the presence of m_4-receptor mRNA on Northern blotting (72) and a preponderance of M_4-receptor protein (73). In situ hybridization has demonstrated that this M_4-receptor mRNA is localized to alveolar walls, and vascular and airway smooth muscle (28). In human lung Northern analysis has not revealed any evidence of either m_4- or m_5-receptor mRNA, and in situ hybridization has not revealed any evidence for expression of the genes for these receptor subtypes (6).

VI. Clinical Relevance of Muscarinic Receptor Subtypes

The discovery of at least three muscarinic subtypes in lung has important clinical implications, since it raises the possibility of more selective anticholinergic therapy in the future. Atropine, ipratropium bromide, and oxitropium bromide are nonselective as anticholinergic drugs and therefore block prejunctional (M_2) and postjunctional (M_3) receptors. Inhibition of the autoreceptor means that more acetylcholine will be released during cholinergic nerve stimulation, and this may overcome postjunctional blockade, thus making these nonselective antagonists less efficient than a selective antagonist of M_3 receptors. Direct evidence for this is the increase in acetylcholine release on nerve stimulation that occurs in the presence of atropine (74), and the fact that ipratropium bromide in low doses causes an increase in vagally mediated bronchoconstriction (38) and increases acetylcholine release from human airways in vitro (44). A similar analogy exists with α-adrenoceptors and the nonselective antagonist phentolamine, by acting on a prejunctional $α_2$-receptor, increases noradrenaline release and is thus far less effective in the treatment of high blood pressure than a selective $α_1$-antagonist such as prazosin, which acts only on the postjunctional receptor. Unfortunately, muscarinic drugs with the high selectivity shown by prazosin for postjunctional receptors are not yet available.

Blockade of muscarinic autoreceptors by drugs such as ipratropium bromide might account for some of the cases of paradoxical bronchoconstriction after inhaled anticholinergic drugs in patients with COPD (75). Presumably anticholinergic drugs selective for M_3 receptors may be more effective and should not have the same risk of precipitating paradoxical bronchoconstriction.

The demonstration of different muscarinic receptor subtypes in airways may have important clinical implications. Further elucidation of the physiological role for these receptor subtypes will depend on the development of more selective antagonists. Drugs such as methoctramine, which have a high degree of selectivity for M_2 receptors, are promising tools for elucidation of the role of muscarinic receptor subtypes, but drugs with a higher selectivity for M_3 receptors are likely to be most useful clinically in airway disease. Active efforts are under way to develop such selective drugs.

It has been difficult to develop M_3-selective antagonists, but darifencin (UK-88,525) is reported to be M_3-selective and is in clinical development (76). An M_1/M_3 selective antagonist, rispenzipine, has also been developed and does not increase acetylcholine release (44), but no clinical studies have been reported. Another M_1/M_3 antagonist revatropate (UK-112,166) is in clinical development as a bronchodilator for COPD (76).

VII. Tiotropium Bromide

Tiotropium bromide (Ba 679), a long-acting muscarinic antagonist, has recently been developed (77). Its quaternary ammonium structure is derived from that of ipratropium bromide. In a series of pharmacological studies tiotropium was shown to be a potent muscarinic receptor antagonist, with a prolonged duration of blockade in guinea pig trachea *in vitro* and after inhalation in dogs *in vivo* (78). In Chinese hamster ovary (CHO) cells transfected with human muscarinic receptor subtype cDNAs, apparent binding affinity (K_D) of tiotropium bromide and ipratropium bromide were similar for hm_1, hm_2, and hm_3 receptors, but kinetic studies (at 23°C) showed that [^{3}H]tiotropium bromide dissociated over 100 times more slowly than [^{3}H]ipratropium bromide from hm_1 (14.6 *vs*. 0.11 h) and hm_3 (34.7 *vs*. 0.26 h), whereas dissociation from hm_2 (0.035 *vs*. 3.6 h) was more similar (78). This suggests that tiotropium bromide has a kinetic selectivity for M_1 and M_3 receptors over M_2 receptors.

A. Binding Studies in Human Lung

[^{3}H]tiotropium bromide binds with high affinity to a uniform population of muscarinic receptors in human peripheral lung membranes (79). The binding affinity of the muscarinic antagonist [^{3}H]N-methyl scopolamine (NMS) was approximately sixfold lower, and competition studies showed that tiotropium bromide was approximately 10-fold more potent than ipratropium bromide and atropine in displacing specific [^{3}H]NMS binding. There is no evidence for selectivity in the binding of [^{3}H]tiotropium bromide to rat cerebral cortex

M_1 receptors labeled with [^{3}H]telenzepine, or heart M_2 and salivary gland M^3 receptors, labeled with [^{3}H]NMS. Tiotropium bromide had a longlasting protective effect against [^{3}H]NMS binding, and this lasted for >90 min, whereas ipratropium bromide had little protective effect. Similarly, [^{3}H]tiotropium bromide dissociates extremely slowly from human lung membranes, with a half-life (at 30°C) of almost 4 h.

Autoradiographic mapping of [^{3}H]tiotropium bromide in human lung sections showed labeling of alveolar walls and submucosal glands, with little specific labeling of airway smooth muscle or epithelium. Both pirenzepine and 4-DAMP displaced specific binding, but methoctramine was without any effect, suggesting that M_1 and M_3 receptors were labeled.

B. Effects on Cholinergic Neurotransmission

Tiotropium bromide potently inhibits cholinergic nerve-induced contraction of guinea pig trachea and is approximately fivefold more potent than ipratropium bromide or atropine (80). The onset of action of tiotropium bromide is slower than that seen with atropine or ipratropium bromide, and after washout, its duration of action in blocking cholinergic neural responses is greatly prolonged, with a $t_{1/2}$ of 540 min, compared with 81 min for ipratropium bromide. In human bronchi tiotropium bromide had a similar inhibitory effect and was 10 times more potent than atropine. Again, the onset of action is slow compared with atropine, and its offset very prolonged ($t_{1/2} > 300$ min) compared to atropine ($t_{1/2}$ 64 min). These studies indicate that tiotropium bromide has a very prolonged inhibitory effect against endogenous ACh released from postganglionic nerve endings in the airways, presumably via an inhibitory effect on postjunctional M_3 receptors.

Electrical field stimulation increases ACh release, measured by a [^{3}H]choline superfusion technique, by approximately sixfold (81). Tiotropium bromide, ipratropium bromide, and atropine all increase ACh release to a similar extent (30% to 40%), but this is lost 2 h after washout of the antagonists. Thus, although tiotropium bromide causes prolonged blockage of airway smooth muscle M_3 receptors after washout, this does not appear to apply prejunctional M_2 autoreceptors. This demonstrates the kinetic selectivity of tiotropium bromide, first demonstrated in binding studies to transfected cells (78), also applies in *in vitro* functional studies.

C. Clinical Studies

The effect of inhaled tiotropium bromide has also been studied in clinical studies in patients with COPD and asthma. In patients with COPD inhaled tiotropium bromide was found to cause a dose-related bronchodilator response which persisted for over 24 h at the highest doses used (82,83). The drug is well tolerated and no significant side effects were reported at single doses of up to 160 µg; in normal volunteers no adverse effects have been reported in doses up to 200µg (78). In asthmatic patients there is also a prolonged bronchodilator effect of inhaled tiotropium bromide. In addition, tiotropium bromide provides prolonged dose-dependent protection against inhaled methacholine challenge (84). At an inhaled dose of 40 µg there is a protection of over seven doubling dilutions against methacholine, and protection lasted for 48 h. This should be compared with a protective effect of oxitropium bromide of < 6 h (85). There were no adverse effects of inhaled tiotropium bromide and no effects on heart rate or blood pressure in these studies.

These clinical studies support the animal and *in vitro* studies and show that tiotropium bromide is a potent and longlasting antimuscarinic agent. It is likely to be a useful addition to the therapy of COPD, where once-daily administration may prove to be more convenient than the currently recommended three- to four-times-daily treatment needed for ipratropium bromide. The prolonged protection against cholinergic neural bronchoconstriction may also be useful in the control of nocturnal asthma, where cholinergic mechanisms appear to be important (86). Whether the kinetic selectivity for M_1 and M_3 receptors over M_2 receptors will be useful clinically remains to be determined. Side effects do not appear to be a problem at doses that are useful clinically, although it will be important to protect against eye contact; a dry powder inhaler formulation rather than a metered dose inhaler may be the most appropriate. Further studies are now indicated looking at more prolonged dosing, and monitoring of effects on airway function and mucus secretion.

VIII. Regulation of Muscarinic Receptor Expression

Despite the fact that muscarinic receptor subtypes have been cloned, there is relatively little information about their regulation at the molecular level. The upstream promoter regions of muscarinic receptors have been difficult to sequence, so there is little information about the transcription factors that may regulate muscarinic receptor expression, although the M_4 receptor promoter region has recently been characterized (87). M_2 receptors have been studied in greatest detail (62). HEL 299 cells are a human embryonic lung fibroblast cell line that expresses M_2 receptors in the absence of M_1 and M_3 receptors, and has therefore been useful for studying regulation of M_2 receptors at the molecular level.

A. Effect of Cholinergic Agonists

Specific [^{3}H]NMS and [^{3}H]QNB binding to muscarinic receptors in HEL 299 cells is best described by the interaction of the radioligands with a single population of high-affinity binding sites. The cholinergic agonist carbachol (1 mM) induces a time-dependent decrease in the number of muscarinic receptors measured with the hydrophilic ([^{3}H]NMS) and the lipophilic ([^{3}H]QNB) ligands without any change in the affinity of the remaining binding sites (88). This suggests that the detected receptor downregulation is due to a decrease in receptor density and not a result of the presence of residual agonist in the binding assay. The loss of the lipophilic [^{3}H]QNB binding sites during the first 2 h of carbachol treatment occurred at slower rate than does the loss of [^{3}H]NMS binding sites as a result of receptor sequestration. Within 12 h, the process had approached steady state with 40% to 60% loss of receptors. The downregulation seen after longterm carbachol treatment is probably due to receptor degradation triggered by prolonged carbachol occupancy. This downregulation is accompanied by uncoupling of the M_2 receptors after 24-h carbachol treatment. These results also suggest that homologous sequestration, desensitization, and downregulation of muscarinic M_2 receptors do not involve transcriptional or posttranscriptional modification of m_2 receptor mRNAs. There was no reduction in either m_2-receptor mRNA stability or m_2-receptor gene transcription measured by nuclear run-on assay (88). This is in contrast to a reduction in m_2-receptor mRNA reported after carbachol incubation in cultured neuronal cells (89).

B. Cross-Talk Between Muscarinic m_2 and β_2-Adrenergic Receptors

HEL 299 cells express functional β_2-adrenergic receptors in HEL 299 cells. The β-adrenergic antagonist [^{125}I]iodopindolol recognizes a single population of binding sites on these cells, and these receptors display characteristic properties of the β_2-adrenoceptor subtype with regard to ligand binding, functional response (cAMP accumulation), and mRNA expression. The presence of functional M_2 and β_2-adrenergic receptors in HEL 299 cells makes it possible to investigate cross-talk between these two receptors. Carbachol (1 mM) treatment has no effect on the density or the affinity of β_2-adrenoceptors in these cells. However, short-term incubation with the long-acting β_2-adrenergic receptor agonist procaterol (5 μM) induces sequestration of the muscarinic receptors followed by their recycling to the cell surface before subsequent downregulation (90). Downregulation was accompanied by functional uncoupling of the M_2 receptors, as inhibition of cAMP accumulation by carbachol was lost after 24-h treatment with procaterol. Downregulation in receptor number was not a consequence of changes in m_2 gene expression, as 24-h procaterol treatment did alter m_2 mRNA levels, although shorter treatments resulted in a modest (25%) but significant increase in m_2 mRNA between 0.5 and 2 h. The loss in receptor density appears to be cAMP-dependent, as it is mimicked by Forskolin and by cAMP analog 8-bromo-cAMP. The cellular kinases, protein kinase A (PKA) and protein kinase C (PKC), are also implicated in the downregulation and desensitization process, as selective inhibitors of both PKA (H-8) and PKC (GF 109203X) fully and partially attenuate downregulation and desensitization, respectively (90).

C. Effect of Protein Kinase C Activation

Direct stimulation of PKC with the phorbol ester phorbol 13, 14-dibutyrate (PDBu: 100 nM) results in a time-dependent decrease in [^{3}H]NMS binding and the steady-state levels of m_2-muscarinic receptor mRNA, and leads to a functional uncoupling of M_2 receptors (91). The loss of m_2-receptor mRNA and protein in HEL 299 cells after exposure to PDBu appears to be a PKC-mediated effect since pretreatment with the PKC inhibitor GF109203X completely inhibits the PDBu-induced reduction in m_2-receptor mRNA and significantly inhibits the reduction in M_2-receptors. Incubation with the inactive 4α-PDBu (100 nM) confirms a PKC-mediated effect, as 24-h treatment had no effect on [^{3}H]NMS binding or m_2-receptor mRNA levels. Potential PKC desensitization following long-term treatment with PDBu is not observed as the calcium ionophore A23187, which is thought to potentiate the effect of PKC stimulation, in combination with PDBu does not produce any further downregulation of M_2 muscarinic receptor protein or mRNA. This result indicates a relative insensitivity of PKC present in HEL 299 to calcium which may relate to a particular PKC isoform in these cells. Elevation of intracellular Ca^{2+} by the ionophore A23187 has no effect on the [^{3}H]NMS binding capacity or on the level of muscarinic m_2 mRNA. This result argues against the involvement of the Ca^{2+}-calmodulin-dependent protein kinase in the downregulation of M_2 receptors.

The reduction in muscarinic m_2-receptor mRNA is not due to posttranscriptional modification of the mRNA but is mediated through a reduction in the rate of transcription of the m_2-receptor gene, as measured by nuclear run-on assays. Furthermore, this downregulation requires protein synthesis, as the translation inhibitor cyclohexamide protects against receptor downregulation. Thus, synthesis of at least one other protein factor is required after PKC stimulation to alter m_2-receptor mRNA levels. The nature of the protein(s) induced by PKC activation is not known. However, PKC is known to phosphorylate and induce DNA binding activity of a number of proteins, including transcription factors such as nuclear factor-κB (NF-κB) and activator protein 1 (AP-1), which may in turn alter the expression of other genes (92,93).

Recently, several interactions have been shown between PKC and mitogen-activated protein (MAP) kinases and in particular the Raf-1-activated pathway that results in the activation of extracellular-signal regulated kinases (ERK1, ERK-2) (94). ERK activation is selectively blocked by the inhibitor PD 098059, which inhibits MAPKK (MEK) (95). This inhibitor partially blocked the phorbol ester reduction in m_2-receptor mRNA, indicating that some of the effects of PKC activation are mediated via MAP kinase and ERK activation (96).

D. Effect of Cytokines and Growth Factors

Transforming growth factor-β (TGF-β) occurs as a group of disulfide-linked proteins comprising 12.5-kDa homodimers which are synthesized and secreted by most cell types as latent high-molecular-weight complexes (97). They exert their action by binding to specific cell surface serine/threonine kinase receptors. TGF-β1 has important physiological roles in the regulation of embryogenesis, tissue repair, inflammation or cell adhesion, growth, and differentiation. In an effort to gain a better understanding of the regulation of muscarinic receptor expression, particularly in inflammatory diseases, we investigated the effect of TGF-β1 on the gene expression of M_2 muscarinic receptors in HEL 299 cells. In human embryonic lung fibroblasts, TGF-β1 induces a time-dependent downregulation of M_2 muscarinic receptor binding sites as measured by [^{3}H]NMS. This downregulation was slow, with 58% loss of total receptors after 24 h of treatment. The affinity of [^{3}H]NMS for the remaining sites was unaltered by TGF-β1. Northern blot analyses showed a 72% decrease in the steady-state levels of m_2 muscarinic receptor mRNA following TGF-β1 treatment for 24 h (98). The loss of [^{3}H]NMS binding sites occurs slowly, which reflects a fall in the steady-state levels of m_2-receptor mRNA, rather than internalization of the receptors through phosphorylation. The delay between protein loss and the fall in mRNA levels may be indicative of the rate of receptor turnover within the cell. The TGF-β1 effect is long-lasting ($t_{1/2} \sim 8$ h) as at least 12 h was required for m_2-receptor mRNA to return to basal levels after TGF-β1 washout. Previous results obtained in the same cell line have shown that the recovery of M_2-receptor protein after receptor alkylation is mainly through the synthetic pathway, with an estimated half-life of receptor synthesis around 12 h (99). The loss in [^{3}H]NMS binding is accompanied by a reduced adenylyl cyclase activity and functional desensitization of M_2 muscarinic receptors. There is no effect of TGF-β1 on the muscarinic m_2-receptor mRNA half-life measured in the presence of actinomycin D, but the rate of m_2-receptor gene transcription measured with nuclear run-on assay was reduced by 50%, indicating reduced gene transcription (98).

There is a requirement for *de novo* protein synthesis for receptor downregulation. The nature of the protein(s) induced by TGF-β1 activation is not known. However, TGF-β1 is known to induce DNA binding activity of a number of proteins, including transcription factors such as AP-1. Electrophoretic DNA mobility shift assays showed a rapid and concomitant increase in AP-1 and NF-κB, but not OCT-1, DNA binding activity to nuclear extracts from cells treated with TGF-β1 stimulation (98). This increase peaked at 15 to 30 min after treatment and declined to control levels thereafter. The antioxidant pyrrolidine dithiocarbamate significantly repressed the induction of NF-κB, but not AP-1, by TGF-β1. The same treatment provided a significant protection against TGF-β1-induced downregulation of M_2-receptor protein and gene expression. These results suggest the involvement, at least in part, of the transcription factor NF-κB in the downregulation process. However, our results do not rule out the involvement of other transcription factors. Indeed, the kinetics of AP-1 and NF-κB induction by TGF-β1 was very rapid, suggesting activation of DNA binding of preexisting molecules rather than the occurrence of *de novo* protein synthesis. On the other hand, the cycloheximide data suggest that there is a requirement for protein synthesis for receptor downregulation. Direct interactions of these transcription factors with the m_2-receptor gene promoter cannot be measured directly, as no sequence data are available to date.

Cytokines released by immune and inflammatory cells infiltrating the airways are well recognized as key mediators in the orchestration and perpetuation of the chronic inflammation in asthma (100). The pro-inflammatory cytokines, tumor necrosis factor α (TNF-α), and interleukin-1β (IL-1β) are increased in asthma. Stimulation of HEL 299 cells with TNF-α or IL-1β had no effect on M_2 muscarinic receptor expression. However, the combination of these two cytokines markedly downregulated muscarinic M_2 receptor protein and uncoupled M_2 receptors from adenylyl cyclase (96). The effect of TNF-α and IL-1β on M_2 muscarinic receptor protein could be extended to mRNA. Whereas downregulation of m_2 muscarinic receptor mRNA is absent in response to either TNF-α or IL-1β alone, there is a dramatic and sustained decrease in downregulation of m_2 mRNA when the two cytokines were administered in combination. The m_2 muscarinic receptor mRNA steadily decreased over time, was apparent after 4 h of stimulation, reached a plateau of 89% control at 14 h, and was stable up to 24 h. There is no effect of TNF-α and

IL-1β on the m_2 muscarinic receptor mRNA stability, and nuclear run-on assays show a reduced m_2 receptor gene transcription. Sequential cytokine addition suggests that the synergy involves postreceptor events.

To characterize the intracellular signaling pathways leading to receptor downregulation, we have investigated the involvement of PKA and PKC in this process. While the PKA inhibitor H-8 provided a significant protection against receptor downregulation, the PKC inhibitor GF109203X had no effect. Beside the classical cyclic AMP and PKC pathways, a third phosphorylation pathways known to be activated by these cytokines is represented by the lipid second-messenger ceramide. IL-1β and TNF-α rapidly increase the cellular content of ceramide produced following the hydrolysis of sphingomyelin by two types of sphingomyelinases—a membrane-associated neutral and an endosomal acidic sphingomyelinase (101). Treatment of HEL 299 cells with N-acetyl-sphingosine (or C2-ceramide), a cell-permeable analog of natural ceramide, did not affect the steady-state levels of m_2 muscarinic receptor mRNA over the time course investigated, in an analogous manner to TNF-α and IL-1β alone. However, the combination of C2-ceramide either with TNF-α or IL-1β markedly downregulated m_2 receptor mRNA expression after 24 h of treatment to a comparable extent to that produced by the combination of the two cytokines. These results are consistent with a role for ceramide pathway in m_2 receptor downregulation induced by the combination of TNF-α and IL-1β treatment.

A further downstream signaling event known to be triggered by TNF-α and IL-1β is activation of the MAP kinase cascade, which comprises the extracellular signal-regulated kinases (ERK) and the c-Jun N-terminal protein kinases (JNK) (94). Using an "in gel kinase assay" we have shown that TNF-α and/or IL-1β activated the JNK-46 and JNK-55 and to a lesser extent p42 and p44 MAP kinase isoforms (96). This result suggests that JNK pathway is preferentially activated by cytokines. These results are in agreement with previous observations showing that the ERK module is primarily activated by mitogenic stimuli whereas JNKs are mainly activated by ceramide, cellular stress such as UV irradiation, and cytokines such as TNF-α and IL-1β (102). However, the absence of synergy between IL-1β and TNF-α at the level of ERKs or JNKs activation suggests that activation of MAP kinases is necessary but not sufficient to cause muscarinic m_2 receptor downregulation. These results suggest that the TNF-α and IL-1β synergize to induce transcriptional downregulation of M_2 muscarinic receptor, which seems to be mediated through activation of both ceramide and PKA pathways. Furthermore, these results suggest that M_2-receptor expression is under the control of a cytokine network.

PDGF also downregulates M_2 receptors in HEL 299 cells, and this appears to be secondary to a fall in m_2 mRNA and reduced gene transcription (103). As with the other cytokines, the reduction in gene transcription is blocked by cyclohexamide and is therefore dependent on the synthesis of some unidentified protein. The PDGF-induced reduction in m_2-receptor mRNA is not accompanied by uncoupling of the remaining receptors, unlike the situation with other cytokines so far investigated, suggesting that PDGF does not result in activation of kinases that phosphorylate muscarinic receptors. PDGF activates several signal transduction pathways with the involvement of multiple kinases. The downregulation of m_2 receptor mRNA was not inhibited by the PKC inhibitor GF 109203X, by the PKA inhibitor H-8, or by the PI-3 kinase inhibitor wortmannin. However, PD 098059 completely blocks the downregulation, indicating that MAPKK and ERKs are involved in the mechanism of downregulation (103).

References

1. Barnes PJ. Muscarinic receptor subtypes in airways. Life Sci 1993; 52:521–528.
2. Hulme EC, Birdsall NJM, Buckley NJ. Muscarinic receptor subtypes. Annu Rev Pharmacol 1990; 30:633–673.
3. Barnes PJ. Muscarinic receptors in airways: recent developments. J Appl Physiol 1990; 68:1777–1785.
4. Minette PA, Barnes PJ. Muscarinic receptor subtypes in airways: function and clinical significance. Am Rev Respir Dis 1990; 141:S162–S165.
5. Maclagan J, Barnes PJ. Muscarinic pharmacology of the airways. Trends Pharmacol Sci 1989; 10(suppl):88–92.
6. Mak JCW, Baraniuk JN, Barnes PJ. Localization of muscarinic receptor subtype mRNAs in human lung. Am J Respir Cell Mol Biol 1992; 7:344–348.
7. Zaagsma J, Roffel AF, Meurs H. Muscarinic control of airway function. Life Sci 1997; 60:1061–1068.
8. Barnes PJ. Neural control of human airways in health and disease. Am Rev Respir Dis 1986; 134:1289–1314.
9. Tokuyama K, Kuo H, Rohde JAL, Barnes PJ, Rogers DF. Neural control of goblet cell secretion in guinea pig airways. Am J Physiol 1990; 259:L108–L115.
10. Barnes PJ, Nadel JA, Roberts JM, Basbaum CB. Muscarinic receptors in lung and trachea: autoradiographic localization using [^{3}H]quinuclidinyl benzilate. Eur J Pharmacol 1982; 86:103–106.
11. Mak JCW, Barnes PJ. Autoradiographic visualization of muscarinic receptor

subtypes in human and guinea pig lung. Am Rev Respir Dis 1990; 141:1559–1568.
12. Van Koppen CJ. Blankenstieijn WM, Klaassen AM, Rodrigues de Miranda JF, Beld AJ, Van Ginneken CAM. Autoradiographic visualization of muscarinic receptors in pulmonary nerves and ganglia. Neursci Lett 1989; 83:237–240.
13. Bloom JW, Halonen M, Lawrence LJ, Rould E, Seaver NA, Yamamura HI. Characterization of high affinity [^{3}H]pirenzepine and ($-$)[H^3]quinuclidinyl benzilate binding to muscarinic receptors in rabbit peripheral lung. J Pharmacol Exp Ther 1987; 240:51–58.
14. Casale TB, Ecklund P. Characterization of muscarinic receptor subtypes in human peripheral lung. J Appl Physiol 1988; 65:594–600.
15. Mak JCW, Barnes PJ. Muscarinic receptor subtypes in human and guinea pig lung. Eur J Pharmacol 1989; 164:223–230.
16. Reinheimer T, Bernedo P, Klapproth H, et al. Acetylcholine in isolated airways of rat, guinea pig, and human: species differences in role of airway mucosa. Am J Physiol 1996; 270:L722–8.
17. Hammer R, Berrie CP, Birdsall NJM, Burgen AS, Hulme EC. Pirenzipine distinguishes between different subclasses of muscarinic receptors. Nature 1980; 283:90–92.
18. Hirschowitz BI, Fong J, Molina E. Effects of pirenzepine and atropine on vagal and cholinergic gastric secretion and gastric release and on heart rate in the dog. J Pharmacol Exp Ther 1983; 225:263–268.
19. Bloom JW, Yamamura HI, Baumgartner C, Halonen M. A muscarinic receptor with high affinity for pirenzepine mediates vagally induced bronchoconstriction. Eur J Pharmacol 1987; 133:21–27.
20. Grandordy BM, Cuss FM, Sampson AS, Palmer JB, Barnes PJ. Phosphatidylinositol response to cholinergic agonists in airway smooth muscle: relationship to contraction and muscarinic receptor occupancy. J Pharmacol Exp Ther 1986; 238:273–279.
21. Madison JM, Jones CA, Tom-Moy M, Brown JR. Affinities of pirenzepine for muscarinic cholinergic receptors in membranes isolated from bovine tracheal mucosa and smooth muscle. Am Rev Respir Dis 1987; 135:719–724.
22. Sertl K, Meryn S, Graninger W, Lagnner A, Schlick W, Ramers H. Acute effects of pirenzepine on bronchospasm. Int J Clin Pharmacol Ther Toxicol 1986; 24:655–657.
23. Cazzola M, Rano S, de Santis D, Principe PJ, Marmo E. Respiratory responses to pirenzepine in healthy subjects. Int J Clin Pharmacol Ther Toxicol 1987; 25 (2):105–109.
24. Ukena D, Wehinger C, Engelstatter R, Steinijans V, Sybrecht GW. The muscarinic M_1-receptor selective antagonist telenzepine has no bronchodilator effects in patients with chronic obstructive airways disease. Eur Resp J 1993; 6:378–382.
25. Lammers J-WJ, Minette P, McCusker M, Barnes PJ. The role of pirenzepine-sensitive (M_1) muscarinic receptors in vagally mediated bronchoconstriction in humans. Am Rev Respir Dis 1989; 139:446–449.

26. Bloom JW, Baumgartener-Folkerts C, Palmer JD, Yamamura HI, Halonen M. A muscarinic receptor subtype modulates vagally stimulated bronchial contraction. J Appl Physiol 1988; 65:2144–2150.
27. Ashe JH, Yarosh CA. Differential and selective antagonism of the slow-inhibitory postsynaptic potential and slow-excitatory postsynaptic potential by gallanin and pirenzepine in the superior cervical ganglion of the rabbit. Neuropharmacology 1984; 23:1321–1329.
28. Mak JCW, Haddad E, Buckley NJ, Barnes PJ. Visualization of muscarinic m_4 mRNA and M_4-receptor subtypes in rabbit lung. Life Sci 1993; 53:1501–1508.
29. Roffel AF, Elzinga CRS, Van Amsterdam RGM, De Zeeuw RA, Zaagsma J. Muscarinic M_2-receptors in bovine trachcal smooth muscle: discrepancies between binding and function. Eur J Pharmacol 1988; 153:73–82.
30. Eglen RM, Hegde SS, Watson N. Muscarinic receptor subtypes and smooth muscle function. Pharmacol Rev 1996; 48:531–565.
31. Yang CM, Chow S, Sung T. Muscarinic receptor subtypes coupled to generation of different second messengers in isolated tracheal smooth muscle cells. Br J Pharmacol 1991; 104:613–618.
32. Fernandes LB, Fryer AD, Hirschman CA. M_2 muscarinic receptors inhibit isoproterenol-induced relaxation of canine airway smooth muscle. J Pharmacol Exp Ther 1992; 262:119–126.
33. Roffel AF, Meurs M, Elzinga CRS, Zaagsma J. Muscarinic M_2 receptors do not participate in the functional antagonism between methacholine and isoprenaline in guinea pig tracheal smooth muscle. Eur J Pharmacol 1993; 249:235–238.
34. Watson N, Magnussen H, Rabe KF. Antagonism of b-adrenoceptor-mediated relaxations of human bronchial smooth muscle by carbachol. Eur J Pharmacol 1995; 275:307–310.
35. Barnes PJ. Modulation of neurotransmission in airways. Physiol Rev 1992; 72:699–729.
36. Faulkner D, Fryer AD, Maclagan J. Post-ganglionic muscarinic inhibitory receptors in pulmonary parasympathetic nerves in guinea-pig. Br J Pharmacol 1986; 88:181–187.
37. Fryer AD, Elbon CL, Kim AL, Xiao HQ, Levey AI, Jacoby DB. Cultures of airway parasympathetic nerves express functional M_2 muscarinic receptors. Am J Respir Cell Mol Biol 1996; 15:716–725.
38. Fryer AD, Maclagan J. Muscarinic inhibitory receptors in pulmonary parasympathetic nerves in the guinea-pig. Br J Pharmacol 1984; 83:973–978.
39. Minette PA, Barnes PJ. Prejunctional inhibitory muscarinic receptors on cholinergic nerves in human and guinea-pig airways. J Appl Physiol 1988; 64:2532–2537.
40. Watson N, Barnes PJ, Maclagan J. Action of methoctramine, a muscarinic M_2-2 receptor antagonist on muscarinic and nicotine cholinoceptors in guinea pig airways in vivo and in vitro. Br J Pharmacol 1992; 105:107–112.

41. Blaber LC, Fryer AD, Maclagan J. Neuronal muscarinic receptors attenuate vagally-induced contraction of feline bronchial smooth muscle. Br J Pharmacol 1985; 86:723–728.
42. Aas P, Maclagan J. Evidence for prejunctional M_2 muscarinic receptors in pulmonary cholinergic nerves in the rat. Br J Pharmacol 1990; 101:73–76.
43. Ito Y, Yoshitomi T. Autoregulation of acetylcholine release from vagus nerve terminals through activation of muscarinic receptors in the dog trachea. Br J Pharmacol 1988; 93:636–646.
44. Patel HJ, Barnes PJ, Takahashi T, Tadjkarimi S, Yacoub MH, Belvisi MG. Characterization of prejunctional muscarinic autoreceptors in human and guinea-pig trachea *in vitro*. Am J Respir Crit Care Med 1995; 152:872–878.
45. Minette PAH, Lammers J, Dixon CMS, McCusker MT, Barnes PJ. A muscarinic agonist inhibits reflex bronchoconstriction in normal but not in asthmatic subjects. J Appl Physiol 1989; 67:2461–2465.
46. Ayala LE, Ahmed T. Is there a loss of a protective muscarinic receptor mechanism in asthma? Chest 1991; 96:1285–1291.
47. Okayama M, Shen T, Midorikawa J, et al. Effect of pilocarpine on propranolol-induced bronchoconstriction in asthma. Am J Respir Crit Care Med 1994; 149:76–80.
48. Barnes PJ. Muscarinic autoreceptors in airways: their possible role in airway disease. Chest 1989; 96:1220–1221.
49. Barnes PJ. Muscarinic receptor subtypes: implications for lung disease. Thorax 1989; 44:161–167.
50. Ind PW, Dixon CMS, Fuller RW, Barnes PJ. Anticholinergic blockade of beta-blocker induced bronchoconstriction. Am Rev Respir Dis 1989; 139:1390–1394.
51. Fryer AD, Fakahany EE, Jacoby DB. Parainfluenza virus type I reduces the affinity of agonists for muscarinic receptors in guinea-pig lung and heart. Eur J Pharmacol 1990; 181:51–58.
52. Fryer AD, Jacoby DB. Parainfluenza virus infection damages inhibitory M_2-muscarinic receptors on pulmonary parasympathetic nerves in the guinea pig. Br J Pharmacol 1991; 102:267–271.
53. Gies J, Landry Y. Sialic acid is selectively involved in the interaction of agonists M_2 muscarinic acetylcholine receptors. Biochem Biophys Res Commun 1988; 150:673–680.
54. Fryer AD, Wills-Karp M. Dysfunction of M_2-muscarinic receptors in pulmonary parasympathetic nerves after antigen challenge. J Appl Physiol 1991; 71:2255–2261.
55. Ten Berge RE, Krikke M, Teisman AC, Roffel AF, Zaagsma J. Dysfunctional muscarinic M_2 autoreceptors in vagally induced bronchoconstriction of conscious guinea pigs after the early allergic reaction. Eur J Pharmacol 1996; 318:131–139.
56. Elbon CL, Jacoby DB, Fryer AD. Pretreatment with an antibody to interleukin-5 prevents loss of pulmonary M_2 muscarinic receptor function in antigen-challenged guinea pigs. Am J Respir Cell Mol Biol 1995; 12:320–328.
57. Costello RW, Schofield BH, Kephart GM, Gleich GJ, Jacoby DB, Fryer AD.

Localization of eosinophils to airway nerves and effect on neuronal M_2 muscarinic receptor function. Am J Physiol 1997; 273:L93–103.
58. Fryer AD, Costello RW, Yost BL et al. Antibody to VLA-4, but not to L-selectin, protects neuronal M_2 muscarinic receptors in antigen-challenged guinea pig airways. J Clin Invest 1997; 99:2036–2044.
59. Jacoby DB, Gleich GJ, Fryer AD. Human eosinophil major basic protein is an endogenous allosteric antagonist at the inhibitory muscarinic M_2 receptor. J Clin Invest 1993; 91:1314–1318.
60. Evans CM, Fryer AD, Jacoby DB, Gleich GJ, Costello RW. Pretreatment with antibody to eosinophil major basic protein prevents hyperresponsiveness by protecting neuronal M_2 muscarinic receptors in antigen-challenged guinea pigs. J Clin Invest 1997; 100:2254–2262.
61. Gambone LM, Elbon CL, Fryer AD. Ozone-induced loss of neuronal M_2 muscarinic receptor function is prevented by cyclophosphamide. J Appl Physiol 1994; 77:1492–1499.
62. Barnes PJ, Haddad E, Rousell JA. Regulation of muscarinic M_2-receptors. Life Sci 1997; 60:1015–1021.
63. Chilvers ER, Barnes PJ, Nahorski SR. Characterisation of agonist-stimulated incorporation of [^{3}H]myo-inositol into inositol phospholipids and [^{3}H]inositol phosphate formation in guinea pig tracheal smooth muscle. Biochem J 1989; 262:739–746.
64. Roffel AF, Elzinga CRS, Zaagsma J. Muscarinic M_3-receptors mediate contraction of human central and peripheral airway smooth muscle. Pulm Pharmacol 1990; 3:47–51.
65. Chilvers ER, Challiss RAJ, Barnes PJ, Nahorski SR. Mass changes of inositol (1,4,5)trisphosphate in trachealis muscle following agonist stimulation. Eur J Pharmacol 1989; 164:587–590.
66. Okayama M, Mullol J, Baraniuk JN, et al. Muscarinic receptor subtypes in human nasal mucosa: characterization, autoradiographic localization, and function in vitro. Am J Respir Cell Mol Biol 1993; 8:176–187.
67. Ramnarine SI, Haddad EB, Khawaja AM, Mak JC. Rogers DF. On muscarinic control of neurogenic mucus secretion in ferret trachea. J Physiol (Lond) 1996; 494:577–586.
68. Baraniuk JN, Kaliner MA, Barnes PJ. Muscarinic M_3-receptor mRNA in in situ hybridization in human nasal mucosa. Am J Physiol 1992; 6:145–148.
69. Matran R, Alving K, Martling C, Lacroix JS, Lundberg JM. Vagally mediated vasodilatation by motor and sensory nerves in the tracheal and bronchial circulation of the pig. Acta Physiol Scand 1989; 135:29–37.
70. MCormack DG, Mak JC, Minette P, Barnes PJ. Muscarinic receptor subtypes mediating vasodilatation in the pulmonary artery. Eur J Pharmacol 1988; 158: 293–297.
71. Emala CW, Clancy J, Hirshman CA. Glucocorticoid treatment decreases muscarinic receptor expression in canine airway smooth muscle. Am J Physiol 1997; 272:L745–L751.

72. Lazareno S, Buckley NJ, Roberts FF. Characterization of muscarinic M_4 binding sites in rabbit lung, chicken heart and NG 108-15 cells. Mol Pharmacol 1990; 38:805–815.
73. Dorje F, Levey AI, Brann MR. Immunological detection of muscarinic receptor subtype proteins (m1–m5) in rabbit peripheral tissues. Mol Pharmacol 1991; 40:459–462.
74. D'Agostino G, Chiari MC, Grana E, Kilbinger H. Muscarinic inhibition of acetylcholine release from a novel *in vitro* preparation of the guinea pig trachea. Naunyn-Schmiedebergs Arch Pharmacol 1990; 342:141–145.
75. Connolly CK. Adverse reaction to ipratropium bromide. Br Med J 1982; 285: 934–935.
76. Alabaster VA. Discovery and development of selective M_3 antagonists for clinical use. Life Sci 1997; 60:1053–1060.
77. Barnes PJ, Belvisi MG, Mak JCW, Haddad E, O'Connor B. Tiotropium bromide (Ba 679 BR), a novel long-acting muscarinic antagonist for the treatment of obstructive airways disease. Life Sci 1995; 56:853–859.
78. Disse B, Reichal R, Speck G, Travnecker W, Rominger KL, Hammer R. Ba679BR, a novel anticholinergic bronchodilator: preclinical and clinical aspects. Life Sci 1993; 52:537–544.
79. Haddad E, Mak JCW, Barnes PJ. Characterization of [^{3}H]Ba 679, a slow-dissociating muscarinic receptor antagonist in human lung: radioligand binding and autoradiographic mapping. Mol Pharmacol 1994; 45:899–907.
80. Takahashi T, Belvisi MG, Patel H, et al. Effect of Ba 679 BR, a novel long-acting anticholinergic agent, on cholinergic neurotransmission in guinea-pig and human airways. Am J Respir Crit Care Med 1994; 150:1640–1645.
81. Ward JK, Belvisi MG, Fox AJ, et al. Modulation of cholinergic neural bronchoconstriction by endogenous nitric oxide and vasoactive intestinal peptide in human airways in vitro. J Clin Invest 1993; 92:736–743.
82. Maesen FPV, Smeets JJ, Costongs MAL, Wald FDM, Cornelissen PJG BA 679 Br, a new long-acting antimuscarinic bronchodilator; a pilot dose-escalation study. Eur Respir J 1993; 6:1031–1036.
83. Maesen FPV, Smeets JJ, Sledsens TJM, Wald FDM, Cornelissen JPG. Tiotropium bromide, a new long-acting antimuscarinic bronchodilator: a pharmacodynamic study in patients with chronic obstructive pulmonary disease (COPD). Eur Respir J 1995; 6:1506–1513.
84. O'Connor BJ, Towse LJ, Barnes PJ. Prolonged effect of tiotropium bromide on methacholine-induced bronchoconstriction in asthma. Am J Respir Crit Care Med 1996; 154:876–880.
85. Wilson NM, Green S, Coe C, Barnes PJ. Duration of protection by oxitropium bromide against cholinergic challenge. Eur J Respir Dis 1987; 71:455–458.
86. Morrison JFJ, Pearson SB, Dean HG. Parasympathetic nervous system in nocturnal asthma. Br Med J 1988; 296:1427–1429.
87. Wood IC, Roopra A, Harrington C, Buckley NJ. Structure of the m4 cholinergic muscarinic receptor gene and its promoter. J Biol Chem 1995; 270:30933–30940.

88. Haddad E-B, Rousell J, Mak JCW, Barnes PJ. Long-term carbachol treatment-induced down-regulation of muscarinic M_2 receptors but not m_2 receptor mRNA in a human lung cell line. Br J Pharmacol 1995; 116:2027–2032.
89. Fukamauchi F, Saunders PA, Hough C, Chuang D. Agonist-induced down-regulation and antagonist-induced up regulation of m2- and m3- muscarinic acetylcholine receptor mRNA and protein in cultured cerebellar granule cells. Mol Pharmacol 1993; 44:940–949.
90. Rousell J, Haddad E-B, Webb BLJ, Giembycz MA, Mak JCW, Barnes PJ. b-Adrenoceptor-mediated down-regulation of M_2-muscarinic receptors: role of cAMP-dependent protein kinases and protein kinase C. Mol Pharmacol 1996; 49:629–635.
91. Rousell J, Haddad E, Mak JCW, Barnes PJ. Transcriptional down-regulation of m2 muscarinic receptor gene expression in human embrogen lung (HEL 295) cells by protein kinase C. J Biol Chem 1995; 270:7213–7218.
92. Siebenlist U, Franzuso G, Brown R. Structure, regulation and function of NF-KB. Annu Rev Cell Biol 1994; 10:405–455.
93. Pfahl M. Nuclear receptor/AP-1 interaction. Endocrine Rev 1993; 14:651–658.
94. Cobb MH, Goldsmith EJ. How MAP kinases are regulated. J Biol Chem 1995; 270:14843–14846.
95. Alessi DR, Cuenda A, Cohen P, Dudley DT, Saltiel AR. PD 098059 is a specific inhibitor of the activation of mitogen-activated protein kinase kinase in vitro and in vivo. J Biol Chem 1995; 270:27489–27494.
96. Haddad E-B, Rousell J, Lindsay MA, Barnes PJ. Synergy between TNF-a and IL-1b in inducing down-regulation of muscarinic M_2 receptor gene expression. J Biol Chem 1996; 271:32586–32592.
97. Massague J, Attasano L, Wrana JL. The TGF-b family and its composite receptors. Trends Cell Biol 1994; 4:172–178.
98. Haddad E-B, Rousell J, Mak JCW, Adcock IM, Barnes PJ. Transforming growth factor-b1 induces transcriptional down-regulation of the m2 muscarinic receptor gene. Mol Pharmacol 1996; 49:781–787.
99. Haddad E-B, Rousell J, Barnes PJ. Muscarinic M_2 receptor synthesis: study of receptor turnover with propylbenzilylcholine mustard. Eur J Pharmacol Mol Pharmacol Sect 1995; 283:255–258.
100. Barnes PJ. Cytokines as mediators of chronic asthma. Am J Respir Crit Care Med 1994; 150:S42–S49.
101. Kolesnick R, Golde DW. The sphingomyelin pathway in tumor necrosis factor and interleukin-1 signaling. Cell 1996; 77:325–328.
102. Coroneos E, Wang Y, Panuska JR, Templeton DJ, Kester M. Sphingolipid metabolites differentially regulate extracellular signal-regulated kinase and stress-activated protein kinase cascades. Biochem J 1996; 316:13–17.
103. Rousell J, Haddad el-B, Lindsay MA, Barnes PJ. Regulation of m2 muscarinic receptor gene expression by platelet-derived growth factor: involvement of extracellular signal-regulated protein kinases in the down-regulation process. Mol Pharmacol 1997; 52:966–973.

Part Two

APPLIED CLINICAL RESEARCH

3

Anticholinergic Agents as Bronchodilators

NICHOLAS J. GROSS

Loyola University of Chicago
Chicago
and Hines VA Hospital
Hines, Illinois

This chapter provides an overview of the rationale for the use of anticholinergic agents as bronchodilators, available agents, and their actions and roles in clinical allergy practice as it relates to the lower airways.

I. Rationale for Use of Anticholinergic Agents

The rationale for the use of anticholinergic agents is based on the autonomic control of airways function. In the normal human, airways caliber is regulated to a large extent by branches of the autonomic nervous system. The bulk of efferent autonomic nerves in the airways are parasympathetic cholinergic nerves, namely branches of the vagus nerve (1). Their terminals supply the airway smooth muscles and mucous glands predominantly in the central airways. Muscarinic receptors are found in the same territory (2) (see Chap. 2). It might be anticipated, therefore, that cholinergic mechanisms and anticholinergic agents have their predominant effects on large airways, as is the case (see below). Activation of the cholinergic system results in contraction of airway smooth muscle (bronchoconstriction), release of mucus from mucous glands, and probably stimulation of airway mucosal ciliary activity (3,4). These actions are opposed by the sympathetic branch of the autonomic system whose fibers are scant in the human lung (1) and by the nonadrenergic, noncholinergic (NANC) system which is probably mediated through cholinergic nerves.

According to current concepts, resting airways caliber is controlled by bronchomotor tone—a low level of tonic bronchial smooth muscle contraction that permits both dilation and constriction of the airways in response to physiologic demands (3,4). Bronchomotor tone is due in part to cholinergic activity. Both normal subjects and patients with airways disease have cholinergic bronchomotor tone, a fact that is supported by the observation that even normal subjects experience increases in airflow following inhalation of an anticholinergic agent (5). Airways disease may increase the level of bronchomotor tone in both asthma (6) and COPD (7). One rationale for the use of anticholinergic agents in the treatment of obstructive airway diseases, therefore, is that they inhibit ongoing bronchomotor tone and thus increase airflow at all times.

In addition to tonic activity, phasic increases in parasympathetically mediated activity to the airways of both asthmatics and patients with COPD occur in response to a wide variety of physical, chemical, and psychogenic stimuli (3,4,8). Physical stimulation to the lower airways, inhalation of cold dry air, irritant gases and aerosols, allergens, and some inflammatory mediators activate receptors in the airways, sending a train of afferent impulses through afferent vagal fibers to the vagal nuclei, which results in an immediate augmentation of efferent vagal activity and bronchospasm. Although this information has been obtained from a large number of carefully conducted animal studies (3,4), such reflex bronchospastic mechanisms appear to operate in human airways also, as the same responses in humans can be partially or totally inhibited by prior administration of anticholinergic agents. A second rationale for the use of anticholinergic agents, then, is that they protect at least partially against a wide variety of clinically relevant bronchospastic stimuli by limiting reflex cholinergic responses to such stimuli.

II. Cholinergic Muscarinic Receptors in Airways

This subject is discussed in detail in Chapters 2 and 10, but will be briefly reviewed here to provide context for the next section. Acetylcholine, the mediator of parasympathetic activity, is released from the terminal varicosities and nerve endings of parasympathetic fibers in the airway wall. It is the ligand for at least three muscarinic receptor subtypes, called M_1, M_2, and M_3, that are known to be expressed in the lungs (9). The receptor subtype on the airway smooth muscle cells and mucous glands which mediates the typical responses seen in airway diseases are of the M_3 subtype (Fig. 1). Receptors of the M_1 subtype are found in the peribronchial ganglia, where their function is not clear but is likely to promote cholinergic responses and may be related to amplification of the signal transmitted from the pre- to postganglionic fibers. Receptors of the M_2 subtype, in contrast, are located on the postganglionic fibers themselves, and appear to act as autoreceptors. They are believed to provide feedback inhibition to the postganglionic fibers, which limits further release of acetylcholine from these fibers. Activation of these receptors, thus, may be seen as a fine-tuning mechanism that modulates parasympathetically mediated bronchoconstriction and mucus release.

In clinical terms, therefore, this scheme suggests that the undesirable effects of parasympathetic activity in the airways—those one wishes to inhibit with therapy—are due to activation of M_1 and M_3 receptor subtypes. Activity of M_2 receptors is seen as opposition to these and clinically beneficial. Indeed, the bronchoconstriction seen in some pediatric viral infections and allergen exposure has been attributed in part to selective inhibition of M_2 receptors (Chap. 10). All currently available anticholinergic agents inhibit all three muscarinic receptor subtypes. Thus, while they inhibit the M_1 and M_3 receptor subtypes that mediate bronchospasm and mucous secretion, they also inhibit M_2 receptors that modulate these effects. The ideal anticholinergic agent, according to this concept, would be one that was a selective inhibitor of M_1 and M_3 receptor subtypes, but a stimulator of M_2 receptors.

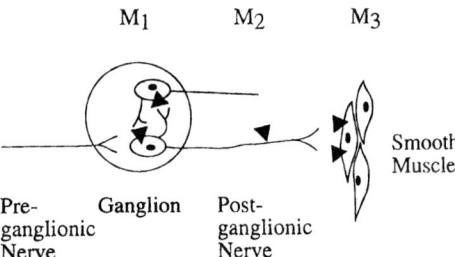

Figure 1 Scheme of the likely location of muscarinic receptor subtypes (black triangles) in airways. M_1, M_2, and M_3 represent the corresponding muscarinic receptor subtypes. (From Ref. 45.)

III. Available and Experimental Anticholinergic Agents

Anticholinergic agents fall into two classes that have distinct pharmacologic properties due principally to the valence of the nitrogen atom on the tropane ring (Fig. 2). In all naturally occurring agents, such as atropine and scopolamine, this nitrogen atom is 3-valent. Tertiary ammonium agents are freely water-soluble and are rapidly and quantitatively absorbed from the skin and mucosal surfaces; they cross the blood brain barrier and are distributed throughout the body. As they inhibit all physiologic parasypathetic activities throughout the body as well as pathologic processes, they result in a wide variety of undesirable systemic side effects.

By contrast, several synthetic agents, some of which closely resemble atropine in structure but in all of which the nitrogen atom is 5-valent have been developed. All such quaternary ammonium agents are synthetic and appear to share the properties of having local anticholinergic activity but being poorly absorbed into the systemic circulation. They can thus be administered in therapeutic doses to the lower respiratory tract without the risks of systemic anticholinergic side effects. Their therapeutic margin is very wide in comparison to atropine (10).

Quaternary agents available in United States include ipratropium bromide (Atrovent), which is available by metered dose inhaler and as a nebulizer solution (11). A combination of ipratropium and albuterol (Combivent) is also available by metered dose inhaler and approved for use in COPD (12,13).

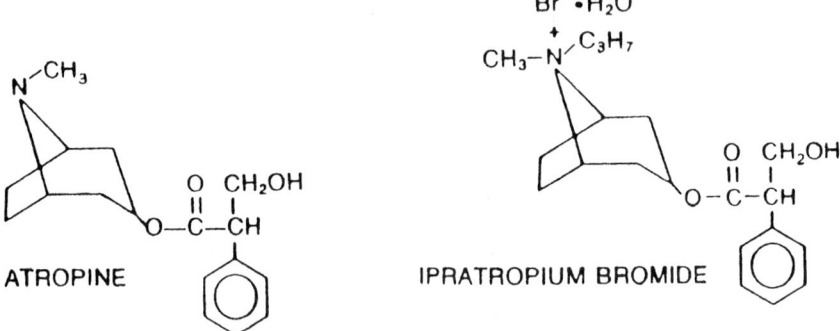

Figure 2 Structures of atropine, a tertiary ammonium compound, and ipratropium, a quaternary compound, to show the charged tropane-ring nitrogen that accounts for many of the pharmacologic properties of ipratropium and related anticholinergic agents.

Glycopyrrolate bromide (Robinul) is a distantly related quaternary anticholinergic agent developed many years ago for the treatment of peptic ulcers, but which has more recently been studied in COPD. Not approved for use in respiratory disease, the injectable form can be administered as an inhalation and appears to have a prolonged action (14). Oxitropium bromide (Oxivent) is closely related to ipratropium but has a slightly longer duration of action. It has been released in Europe but not in the United States. Atropine methonitrate is also closely related to ipratropium and appears to be similar in action (15), but has not been approved for general use in United States. Tiotropium bromide is the first quaternary anticholinergic agent to result from molecular modeling. It is of particular interest in that it is functionally specific for M_1 and M_3 receptor subtypes but not M_2 receptors, which is a desirable combination of pharmacologic properties. It is also very long-acting—possibly longer than 30 hours (16,17). Not yet approved for general use, it offers considerable promise in the management of stable COPD.

IV. Features of Anticholinergic Bronchodilator Actions

A. Site of Action

Anticholinergic agents act at sites in the airways where cholinergic nerves and muscarinic receptors terminate, namely the central airways (2). Physiologic studies tend to confirm that their physiologic effects are mainly on the larger airways (18,19). By contrast, adrenergic agents tend to act on medium-size and smaller airways, where their receptors are concentrated (2). This suggests that anticholinergic and adrenergic agents may complement each other, providing a rationale for their use in combination.

B. Physiologic Actions

Ipratropium and atropine methonitrate, in optimal inhaled doses, typically increase FEV_1 in normal adults by 0.15 L and in patients with COPD by 0.2 to 0.5 L. Like other bronchodilators, they simultaneously decrease lung volumes in patients with COPD (15). But, unlike adrenergic agents, they have minimal effects on pulmonary blood flow and ventilation-perfusion ratios. Thus, they tend not to reduce arterial PO_2 levels, unlike adrenergic agents (20,21). This difference might be a consideration in the selection of a bronchodilator for exacerbations of airways disease. Commensurate with the increase in FEV_1, anticholinergic agents increase effort tolerance (22,23) but probably not more than do adrenergic agents.

C. Onset and Duration of Bronchodilatation

Although their onset of action occurs within minutes, anticholinergic agents typically require 30 min to reach peak effect (24), and often longer. In contrast, adrenergic agents have a very rapid onset of action and reach peak effect within 5 to 15 min (Fig. 3). An adrenergic agent—e.g., albuterol, terbutaline, or metaproterenol—is thus more appropriate for the rapid relief of acute bronchospasm. The duration of bronchodilatation defined as the time FEV_1 remains significantly above baseline, is in the region of 3 to 4 for conventional adrenergic agents and slightly longer for ipratropium, maybe 4 to 6h.

D. Tolerance

Regular use of adrenergic agents results in tolerance or tachyphylaxis in some subjects. Although this phenomenon can be demonstrated in the laboratory, it is not felt to be of clinical relevance. A similar phenomenon has often been sought for anticholinergic agents but, with one exception (25), not found. Moreover, there are reasons why anticholinergic agents, being receptor antagonists rather than agonists, would not be expected to induce tolerance (9).

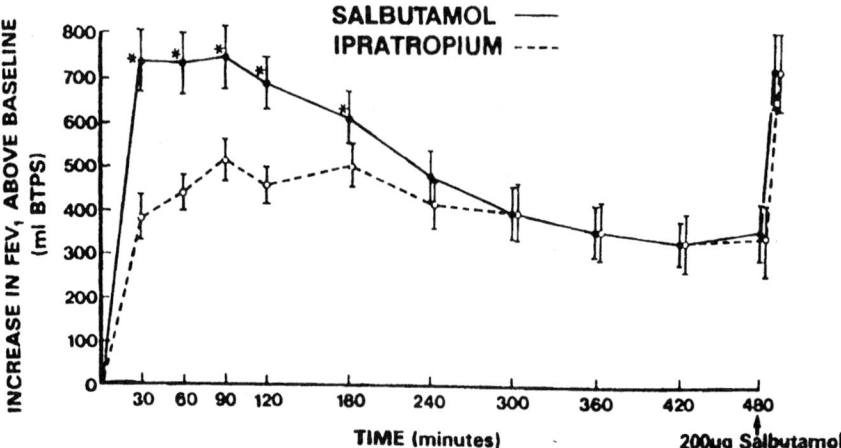

Figure 3 Increase in FEV_1 in 25 patients with asthma after inhalation of 200 µg salbutamol or 40 µg ipratropium (both by metered dose inhaler). All patients received an additional dose of salbutamol at 480 min. Asterisks denote significant differences ($P < .05$). (From Ref. 24.)

V. Clinical Actions

A. Protection Against Bronchospastic Simuli

The protective effect of single doses of an anticholinergic agent have been studied in an attempt to predict whether they might be useful against typical bronchospastic stimuli in the clinical setting. Anticholinergic agents, if given in sufficient dosage, protect completely against the effects of cholinergic agonists such as methacholine or carbachol, as one would expect. Against most other stimuli they provide partial protection at best, and usually less protection than the beta-2 adrenergic agent.

This is interpreted as indicating that stimuli such as histamine, allergen inhalation, and cold dry air produce bronchodilatation by a variety of mechanisms—by direct actions of the airway mucosa and smooth muscle, by the release of mediators from inflammatory cells, by neural reflex mechanisms. Only the last are amenable to anticholinergic inhibition. Overall, therefore, their protection is incomplete, and usually less than that resulting from an adrenergic agent. This pattern is quite consistent with their limited efficacy in asthmatic patients (see below).

Two exceptions to this scheme deserve mention. Ipratropium is a more effective bronchodilator against psychogenic bronchospasm (26,27) presumably because this stimulus is conducted along neural pathways and against the bronchospasm induced by administration of a beta-2 blocking agent (28). When acute bronchospasm is caused by inadvertent administration of a beta-blocking agent to a patient with, for example, unrecognized airways disease, an anticholinergic agent may be the only bronchodilator capable of reversing the bronchospasm.

B. In Asthma

In clinical trials, of which many have been published, anticholinergic agents almost invariably produced modest bronchodilatation in patients with stable asthma but have almost invariably been found to be less potent and slower-acting than beta-agonists (Fig. 3). This can be interpreted as being due to the fact that the airways obstruction of asthma has many mechanisms, which include mucosal edema and hyperemia, mucus in the airway lumen, and smooth muscle contraction. Only the last is affected by an anticholinergic agent, whereas adrenergic agents may temporarily reverse many of the other mechanisms as well as smooth muscle contraction.

Consequently anticholinergic agents do not have a major role in the management of bronchospasm in asthmatics and have not been approved for this use in United States. However, among asthmatics there is considerable variation in the response to anticholinergic agents; some patients in fact respond quite well to them. Nor has it been possible to predict which asthmatics will respond to anticholinergic bronchodilators. Therefore their use may be explored as adjunctive bronchodilators in individual asthmatic patients who are difficult to control despite optimal use of adrenergic agents.

Anticholinergic agents probably also have an adjunctive role in status asthmaticus. In well-controlled studies (e.g., 29), the combination of ipratropium with a beta agonist resulted in greater bronchodilation than did a beta agonist alone. Moreover, the benefit of adding ipratropium was greater in patients with more severe bronchospasm. Meta-analysis of several comparable studies suggests, also, that the addition of ipratropium to adrenergic therapy improves the short-term course of status asthmaticus (30). It is therefore appropriate to use combinations of both classes of agents in the initial management of acute severe asthma, particularly when airflow obstruction is severe. Anticholinergic agents should not be used as monotherapy in status asthmaticus.

C. In Pediatric Asthma

Two consensus reports suggested that ipratropium was safe in stable pediatric asthma but that its benefit was not established (31,32). As in adults, ipratropium may be useful as an adjunct to beta-agonist therapy of acute severe asthma (33).

D. In COPD

Patients with COPD have traditionally be considered, by definition, to be nonresponsive to bronchodilators. This is now known to be incorrect (34). Although patients with COPD probably have less variability in airflow than do patients with asthma and respond less in absolute airflow to bronchodilators, nearly all do manifest some response. As their airflow obstruction is generally much more severe than that of asthmatics, even small increases in absolute airflow may provide significant relief of symptoms. In addition, bronchodilatation may be associated with reduction in static lung volumes (15), which may itself result in symptomatic relief that is not reflected by FEV_1 changes.

A few large studies (e.g., 35) and many smaller studies (Fig. 4) show that an anticholinergic agent consistently results in greater bronchodilatation than any of a variety of adrenergic agents in stable COPD. This experience contrasts with numerous studies in asthmatic patients where an adrenergic agent has consistently been found to be more potent (see above). The difference in the response of asthmatic and COPD patients is illustrated in Figure

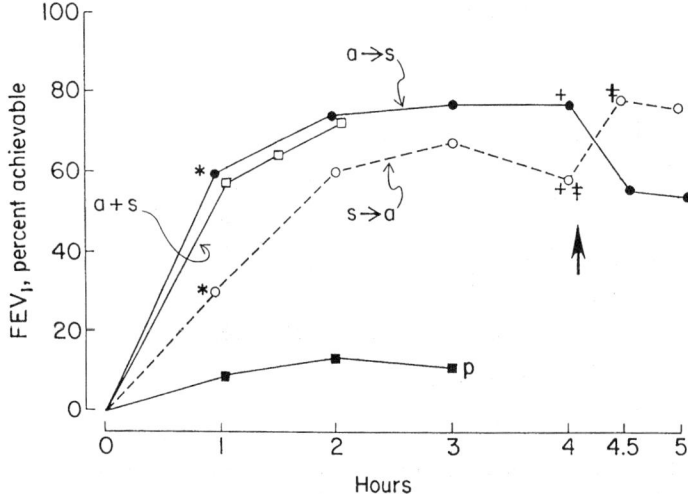

Figure 4 Responses of 10 patients with emphysema to atropine methonitrate (a) and albuterol (s) in sequences. a → s, four doses of atropine methonitrate at hourly intervals followed by albuterol at the arrow; s → a, the same agents in reverse order; a + s, both agents simultaneously; p, placebo. Pairs of symbols indicate significant differences between values. (From Ref. 15.)

5, which is representative of several studies that have compared the responses of patients with asthma and COPD. While the two groups of patients respond approximately equally to ipratropium, asthmatics respond much better to adrenergic agents than do patients with COPD. Consequently, the anticholinergic agent emerges as the more potent bronchodilator in COPD in contrast to asthma.

The interpretation of this result is that airflow limitation in COPD is mainly due to structural mechanisms such as loss of recoil forces and remodeling of the airway wall and that the only reversible component of their airflow obstruction is inhibition of bronchomotor tone, which is largely due to cholinergic activity and therefore best relieved by an anticholinergic agent. This contrasts with the multiple mechanisms of airflow obstruction in asthma, many of which are amenable to adrenergic but not anticholinergic therapy. Whether this explanation is correct or not, anticholinergic agents appear as the more potent bronchodilators in COPD and are currently regarded as first-line bronchodilators in this condition (37–39), in contrast to asthma, where adrenergic agents are clearly more potent.

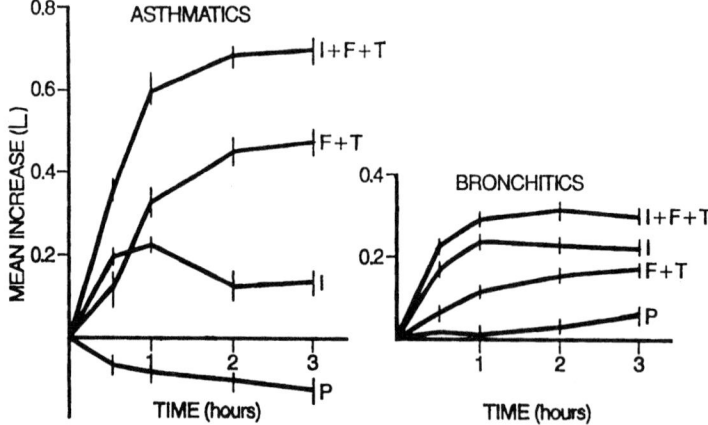

Figure 5 Increase of FEV_1 in 15 patients with asthma (left panel) and 15 patients with chronic bronchitis (right panel). P, placebo; I, ipratropium 40 μg by metered dose inhaler; F + T, fenoterol 5 mg by metered dose inhaler plus oxtriphylline 400 mg oral. (From Ref. 36.)

In acute exacerbations of COPD, no significant differences have emerged between the different classes of bronchodilators (21,29,40).

E. Long-Term Effects

Anticholinergic agents are approved and used as short-term bronchodilators for the temporary relief of symptoms. Evidence that they have long-term effects is less well substantiated. When given over a 5-year period to patients with preclinical COPD, ipratropium did not alter the age-related decline in lung function (41) but did result in a modest increase in FEV_1, which was lost within 2 weeks of its discontinuation. A retrospective analysis of seven large clinical trials showed that baseline (prebronchodilator) FEV_1 and FVC increased (by 28 and 131 mL, respectively) following 90 days of regular administration of ipratropium in usual dosage. No improvement in baseline airflow was observed in patients who had received the alternative, beta-agonist treatment. In addition, the acute response to ipratropium was increased, although by a very small amount, at the end of 90 days' administration, while the acute response to the beta-agonist declined (42).

These two reports raise the possibility that long-term ipratropium treatment might have beneficial effects on airflow that extend days or longer beyond the 4 to 6-hour acute bronchodilator effect. Any long-term improvement was quite modest in these studies and will need further confirmation; however, these reports suggest possible small long-term benefits.

VI. Side Effects

As discussed above, anticholinergic agents fall into two classes, the natural tertiary ammonium agents such as atropine which are well absorbed, and the synthetic quaternary ammonium agents (such as ipratropium) which are poorly absorbed. Atropine and its natural congeners have a very narrow therapeutic margin and cause many side effects such as dry mouth and eyes, hotness and flushing of the skin, palpitations, and tachycardia in the dosage required to produce bronchodilation. Although not serious, these side effects are not well tolerated over the long term. At only slightly higher doses, blurred vision, retention of urine, irritability, and confusion may occur. Atropine should not be given to patients at risk for narrow-angle glaucoma or prostatism. Moreover it may inhibit mucociliary clearance in the airways, and there is also the risk of occasional more serious side effects such as psychosis in older patients. For these reasons atropine and its natural congeners such as scopolamine must now be regarded as obsolete in the management of COPD.

In contrast, the synthetic quaternary ammonium agents are poorly absorbed and pose neglibile risks of systemic side effects. Ipratropium, unlike atropine, can be safely administered to patients with narrow-angle glaucoma or prostatic hypertrophy (11). Nor does it adversely affect mucociliary clearance (43), hemodynamics (44), or gas exchange (20). Massive, accidental overdose of the closely related agent atropine methylnitrate was well tolerated in one patient (10). Following two decades of widespread clinical usage, the newer anticholinergic agents appear to be free of serious side effects.

References

1. Richardson JB. Innervation of the lung. Eur J Respir Dis 1982; 117(suppl):13–31.
2. Barnes PJ, Basbaum CB, Nadel JA. Autoradiographic localization of autonomic receptors in airway smooth muscle, marked differences between large and small airways. Am Rev Respir Dis 1983; 127:758–763.
3. Widdicombe JG. The parasympathetic nervous system in airways disease. Scand J Respir Dis 1979; 103(suppl):38–43.
4. Nadel JA. Autonomic regulation of airway smooth muscle. In: Nadel JA, ed.

Physiology and Pharmacology of the Airways. New York: Marcel Dekker, 1980: 217–257.
5. Gross NJ, Skorodin MS. Anticholinergic agents. In: Jenne JW, Murphy S, eds. Drug Therapy for Asthma, Lung Biology in Health and Disease. Vol. 31. New York: Marcel Dekker, 1987:615–668.
6. Shah PKD, Lakhotia M, Mehta S, Jain SK, Gupta GL. Clinical dysautonomia in patients with bronchial asthma, study with seven autonomic function tests. Chest 1990; 98:1408–1413.
7. Gross NJ, Co E, Skorodin MS. Cholinergic bronchomotor tone in COPD, estimates of its amount in comparison to normal. Chest 1989; 96:984–987.
8. Gross NJ, Skorodin MS. Anticholinergic, antimuscarinic bronchodilators. Am Rev Respir Dis 1984; 129:856–870.
9. Gross NJ, Barnes PJ. A short tour around the muscarinic receptor. Am Rev Respir Dis 1988; 138:765–767.
10. Gross NJ, Skorodin MS. Massive overdose of atropine methonitrate with only slight untoward effects. Lancet 1985; 2:386.
11. Gross NJ. Ipratropium bromide. N Engl J Med 1988; 319:486–494.
12. Petty TL. In chronic obstructive pulmonary disease, a combination of ipratropium and albuterol is more effective than either agent alone: an 85-day multicenter study. Chest 1994; 105:1411–1419.
13. Ikeda A, Nishimura K, Koyama H, Izumi T. Bronchodilating effects of combined therapy with clinical dosages of ipratropium bromide and salbutamol for stable COPD: comparison with ipratropium bromide alone. Chest 1995; 107:401–405.
14. Walker FB, Kaiser DL, Kowal MB, Suratt PM. Prolonged effect of inhaled glycopyrrolate in asthma. Chest 1987; 91:49–51.
15. Gross NJ, Skorodin MS. Role of the parasympathetic system in airway obstruction due to emphysema. N Engl J Med 1984; 311:421–426.
16. O'Connor BJ, Towse LJ, Barnes PJ. Prolonged effect of tiotropium bromide on methacholine-induced bronchoconstriction in asthma. Am J Respir Crit Care Med 1996; 154:876–880.
17. Maesen FP, Smeets JJ, Sledsens TJ, Wald FD, Cornelissen PJ. Tiotropium bromide, a new long-acting antimuscarinic bronchodilator: a pharmacodynamic study in patients with chronic obstructive pulmonary disease (COPD). Eur Respir J 1995; 8: 1506–1513.
18. Ingram RH, Wellman JJ, McFadden ER, Mead J. Relative contributions of large and small airways to flow limitation in normal subjects before and after atropine and isoproterenol. J Clin Invest 1977; 59:696–703.
19. McFadden ER, Ingram RH, Haynes RL, Wellman JJ. Predominant site of airflow limitation and mechanisms of postexertional asthma. J Appl Physiol 1977; 42: 746–752.
20. Gross NJ, Bankwala Z. Effects of an anticholinergic bronchodilator on arterial blood gases of hypoxemic patients with COPD. Am Rev Respir Dis 1987; 136: 1091–1094.
21. Karpel JP, Pesin J, Greenberg D, Gentry E. A comparison of the effects of ipra-

tropium bromide and metaproterenol sulfate in acute exacerbations of COPD. Chest 1990; 98:835–839.
22. Hay JG, Stone P, Carter J, et al. Bronchodilator reversibility, exercise performance and breathlessness in stable chronic obstructive pulmonary disease. Eur Respir J 1992; 5:659–664.
23. Ikeda A, Nishimura K, Koyama H, Sugiura N, Izumi T. Oxitropium bromide improves exercise performance in patients with COPD. Chest 1994; 106:1740–1745.
24. Ruffin RE, Fitzgerald JD, Rebuck AS. A comparison of the bronchodilator activity of Sch 1000 and salbutamol. J Allergy Clin Immunol 1977; 59:136–141.
25. Vaughan TR, Bowen RE, Goodman DL, Weber RW, Nelson HS. The development of subsensitivity to atropine methylnitrate, a double-blind, placebo-controlled crossover study. Am Rev Respir Dis 1988; 138:771–774.
26. McFadden ER, Luparello T, Lyons HA, Bleeker E. The mechanism of action of suggestion in the induction of acute asthma attacks. Psychosom Med 1969; 31:134–143.
27. Rebuck AS, Marcus HI. Sch1000 in psychogenic asthma. Scand J Respir Dis 1979; 103 (suppl):186–190.
28. Grieco MH, Pierson RN. Mechanism of bronchoconstriction due to beta-adrenergic blockade. J Allergy Clin Immunol 1971; 48:143–152.
29. Rebuck AS, Chapman KR, Abboud R, et al. Nebulized anticholinergic and sympathomimetic treatment of asthma and chronic obstructive airways disease in the emergency room. Am J Med 1987; 82:59–64.
30. Ward MJ. The role of anticholinergic drugs in acute asthma. In: NJ Gross, ed. Anticholinergic Therapy in Obstructive Airways Disease. Londor: Franklin Scientific Publications, 1993; 155–162.
31. Warner JO, Getz M, Landau LI, et al. Management of asthma: a consensus statement. Arch Dis Child 1989; 64:1065–1079.
32. Hargreave FE, Dolovich J, Newhouse MT. The assessment and treatment of asthma: a conference report. J Allergy Clin Immunol 1990; 85:1098–1112.
33. Schuh H, Johnson DW, Callahan S, Canny G, Levinson H. Efficacy of frequent nebulized ipratropium bromide added to frequent high-dose albuterol therapy in severe childhood asthma. J Pediatr 1995; 126:639–645.
34. Gross NJ. COPD: a disease of reversible airways obstruction. Am Rev Respir Dis 1986; 133:725–726.
35. Tashkin DP, Ashutosh K, Bleeker E, et al. Comparison of the anticholinergic ipratropium bromide with metaproterenol in chronic obstructive pulmonary disease, a 90 day multicenter study. Am J Med 1986; 81 (suppl 5A):81–86.
36. Lefcoe NM, Toogood JH, Blennerhassett G, Patterson NAM. The addition of an aerosol anticholinergic to an oral beta agonist plus theophylline in asthma and bronchitis. Chest 1982; 82:300–305.
37. Ferguson GT, Cherniack RM. Management of chronic obstructive pulmonary disease. N Engl J Med 1993; 328:1017–1022.
38. Siafakis NM, Vermiere P, Pride NB, et al. ERS consensus statement: optimal

assessment and management of chronic obstructive pulmonary disease. Eur Respir J 1995; 8:1398–1420.
39. ATS Statement. Standards for the diagnosis and care of patients with chronic obstructive pulmonary disease. Am J Respir Crit Care Med 1995; 152:S77–S120.
40. Patrick DM, Dales RE, Stark RM, Laliberte G, Dickinson G. Severe exacerbations of COPD and asthma, incremental benefit of adding ipratropium to usual therapy. Chest 1990; 98:295–297.
41. Anthonisen NR, Connett JE, Kiley JP. Effects of smoking intervention and the use of an inhaled anticholinergic bronchodilator on the rate of decline of FEV_1: the Lung Health Study. JAMA 1994; 272:1497–1505.
42. Rennard SI, Serby CW, Ghafouri M, Johnson PA, Friedman M. Extended therapy with ipratropium is associated with improved lung function in patients with COPD, a retrospective analysis of data from seven clinical trials. Chest 1996; 110:62–70.
43. Pavia D, Bateman JRM, Sheehan NF, Clarke SW. Effect of ipratropium bromide on mucociliary clearance and pulmonary function in reversible airways obstruction. Thorax 1979; 34:501–507.
44. Chapman KR, Smith DL, Rebuck AS, Leenen FHH. Hemodynamic effects of inhaled ipratropium bromide alone and in combination with an inhaled $beta_2$-agonist. Am Rev Respir Dis 1983; 132:845–847.
45. Gross NJ. Anticholinergic agents. In: AR Leff, ed. Pulmonary and Critical Care Pharmacology and Therapeutics. New York: McGraw-Hill, 1996, p. 535.

4

Anticholinergic Drug Therapy in the Management of Acute Severe Asthma

JEFFREY E. GARRETT

Green Lane Hospital
Auckland, New Zealand

I. Introduction

International guidelines on acute asthma management endorse inhaled bronchodilator therapy, supplemental oxygen, and systemic corticosteroids (1–3). Beta-agonists are the recommended initial bronchodilator, and the severity of the attack determines whether they are delivered by nebulizer or by an MDI with spacer. Response to initial therapy should determine both the subsequent dose and the frequency of administration of beta-agonist therapy. Two recent studies in acute severe asthma (4,5) suggest a greater improvement over 2 hours when inhaled beta-agonists are administered continuously than when administered intermittently. While the majority of patients respond to this treatment approach, the degree of response, the amount of bronchodilator therapy consumed previously during the attack, and the severity of attack will determine whether other bronchodilators are likely to be efficacious and whether the inhaled or intravenous approach should be employed. Intravenous theophyllines have generally lost favor, since they infrequently add to the effect of inhaled bronchodilating therapy and since they have such a narrow therapeutic index (6). Toxicity may be induced particularly in the critically ill due to acute changes in hepatic metabolism and drug handling (6). Intravenous beta-agonist therapy has been shown to augment inhaled beta-agonist therapy in very severe attacks, particularly when patients are having difficulty in tolerating nebulized therapy (7). However, unless the attack of asthma is particularly severe and the patient is intolerant of, or unable to be administered, inhaled therapy, then intravenous beta-agonist therapy contributes to improvement in neither lung function nor therapeutic effect (8–10), and causes more side effects.

Anticholinergics have a weaker bronchodilating action than beta-agonists (11,12), but because they may augment the effect of beta-agonists and have few side effects, their place in the management of acute asthma warrants further scrutiny. Acute bronchospasm is associated with increased reflex vagal discharge, and this provides a biologically plausible explanation as to why anticholinergic therapy may augment beta-agonist therapy and why the response to nebulized beta-agonist therapy may be attenuated.

Although atropine methonitrate and atropine sulfate have been shown to augment the effect of beta-agonists in acute asthma (13), they have been superseded by ipratropium bromide, a quaternary derivative of atropine. In high doses ipratropium produces bronchodilatation without the local effects of dry mouth and sputum retention which complicate the use of atropine. This review will therefore concentrate solely on ipratropium and will address the following questions.

In the management of asthma exacerbations:

What is the optimal dose of nebulized ipratropium bromide?
Does inhaled ipratropium bromide augment the effect of beta-agonist therapy?
Does inhaled ipratropium bromide contribute anything to maximally employed beta-agonist therapy?
Does inhaled ipratropium bromide contribute to improvements in clinical outcome such as a reduction in recovery time, reduced need for other medication, reduced need for hospitalization, or reduction in length of hospital stay?
Is there a pharmacoeconomic argument for use of inhaled ipratropium bromide in acute asthma?
Are there patient subgroups who particularly benefit from anticholinergic therapy?

II. What Is the Optimal Dose of Ipratropium Bromide in Acute Severe Asthma?

In stable asthma, the optimal dose of ipratropium bromide is considered to be 40 to 80 µg (14). However, doses of up to 500 µg may be required in severe asthma, possibly as a result of increased vagal discharge and the fact that nebulizers deliver medication less efficiently to the airways than do MDIs (15). No study has shown any additional short-term benefit in terms of bronchodilator effect or duration of action from doses of >500 µg per dose.

III. Does Inhaled Ipratropium Bromide Augment the Effect of Beta-Agonist Therapy?

Six studies have compared the efficacy of ipratropium bromide alone with nebulized beta-agonist therapy alone. While one study suggested that 500 µg of ipratropium bromide was as effective as 10 mg of salbutamol sulfate (15), none of the other five studies, which employed doses of between 0.625 mg fenoterol and 5 mg salbutamol, showed superior bronchodilation (11,12,15–18). The study numbers employed ranged from 12–100 and were insufficient to overcome a type II error. However, combined analysis showed superior bronchodilation when inhaled beta-agonists alone are compared with ipratropium bromide alone ($P < .05$) (19).

In a pooled analysis of nine randomized trials of treatment of acute exacerbations of asthma reported prior to 1990 (11,12,15–18,20–22), Ward (19) noted significantly more bronchodilatation ($P < .05$) following nebulization with combined ipratropium and beta-agonist therapy than with beta-agonists alone (salbutamol or fenoterol). Although four of the studies (15–17,22) showed a significant advantage from combination therapy ($P < .05$), insufficient sample sizes meant that the potential for a type II error in individual studies was large.

Since 1990 three large randomized studies, in New Zealand, the United States, and Canada (23–25), have been performed to determine whether combination therapy is superior to monotherapy in the treatment of acute asthma. All three studies had large sample sizes to overcome the possibility of type II errors which made evaluation of earlier studies difficult. In the Canadian (25) and New Zealand (23) studies a single dose of ipratropium bromide 0.5 mg and salbutamol 2.5 mg was compared with salbutamol 2.5 mg alone, whereas the U.S. study (24) employed two administrations (one at baseline and the other 45 min later). Unfortunately, these three studies did not conclusively resolve the uncertainty concerning the potential benefits of combination therapy. The U.S. study reported no additional effect on lung function from combination therapy (ΔFEV_1 −17 mL), the Canadian study a small but nonsignificant effect (ΔFEV_1 92 mL) ($P = .08$), and the New Zealand study a significant improvement in lung function (ΔFEV_1 113 mL) among patients receiving combination therapy ($P < .05$). A pooled analysis was subsequently undertaken (26) to assess the effect of combination therapy in general and to evaluate the apparent discrepancies in results from these three studies. The pooled analysis found that combination therapy at the dose administered conferred a small benefit compared with monotherapy (Fig. 1). The difference between the New Zealand and Canadian studies was small, with mean improvement in FEV_1 of 113 mL and 92 mL, respectively. Conversely, the U.S. study showed that patients on combination therapy did worse (−17 mL FEV_1).

In the U.S. study, the mean change in FEV_1 and the median change in FEV_1 pointed in opposite directions. One reason related to a small number of outliers (n = 8) whose FEV_1 increased by more than 2.5 L of whom six received salbutamol monotherapy. Such a large improvement in FEV_1 is unlikely

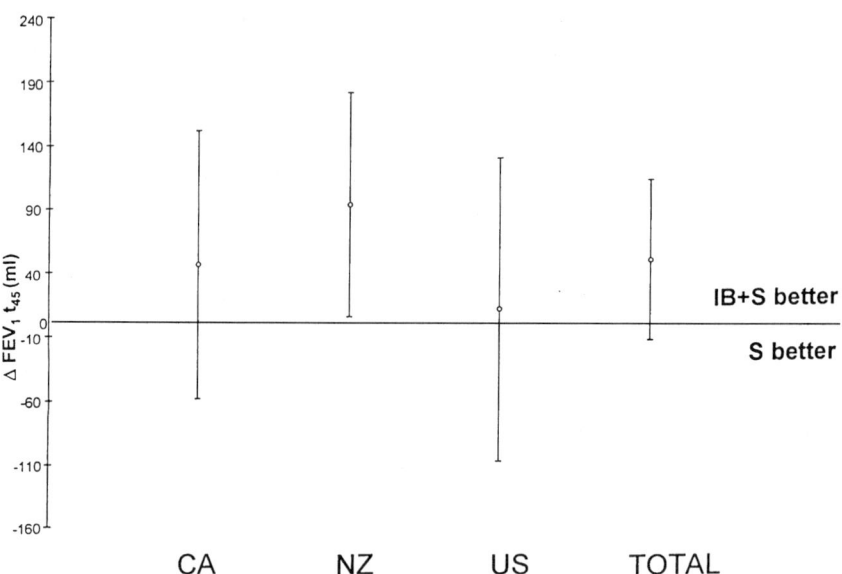

Figure 1 Change in mean FEV_1 at T_{45}.

after a single dose of nebulized bronchodilator and most likely reflects inaccurate measurement of baseline lung function. When these outliers were excluded from the U.S. analysis the mean improvement in FEV_1 was 30 mL in favor of combination therapy (as opposed to -17 mL) (26). Differences in the quality of lung function therefore seemed to explain at least some of the difference among the three studies. In New Zealand, a computerized quality assurance program adapted for use from the North American lung health study (27) contributed to more accurate measurement of FEV_1 with less variation (95% CI for the absolute improvement in FEV_1 20–206, range 186 mL), compared with the Canadian (95% CI -22–206, range 228 mL) and U.S. studies (95% CI -149–115, range 264 mL). The conclusion drawn from the pooled analysis (26) was that there is a small beneficial effect on lung function as a consequence of combination therapy.

IV. Does Inhaled Ipratropium Bromide Contribute Anything to Maximally Employed Beta-Agonist Therapy?

In two studies (16,21) performed prior to 1990, the dose of beta-agonist chosen was thought to have been at the plateau of the dose-response curve. Bryant (17) had previously shown that after initial treatment with 1 mg of nebulized fenoterol, a second dose produced no further improvement but extra benefit was achieved by adding ipratropium. Ward et al. (28) showed that 10 mg of nebulized salbutamol given 2 hours apart produced less bronchodilatation than 10 mg salbutamol and 0.5 mg ipratropium. Thus existing information supports the view that ipratropium does contribute to maximally applied doses of beta-agonist.

Few studies have endeavored to evaluate the influence of prior bronchodilator therapy on the response to inhaled bronchodilator treatment in the emergency room. Rossing et al. (29) have shown no difference in baseline lung function or in response to bronchodilator therapy when those pretreated within the community with beta-agonists were compared with those who were not. However, this study may not have had the power to assess any difference. Janson (30) and Boe (31) found a negative correlation between serum beta-agonist level on arrival at the emergency department and the degree of bronchodilatation after intravenous salbutamol but not after inhaled salbutamol. Conversely, we found that higher baseline salbutamol levels were associated with both more severe asthma at the time of attendance and a poorer response to therapy (32). Further, in patients with serum salbutamol levels above

2 µmole/L or who had consumed <10 puffs of salbutamol MDI or a single nebulizer in the previous 6 hours, there was no added benefit from the addition of ipratropium. Conversely, patients who had taken no beta-agonist therapy exhibited the greatest improvement in lung function with the addition of ipratropium bromide (23). Similar results were noted in the Canadian study (25).

In conclusion, the question as to whether ipratropium bromide contributes anything to maximally applied doses of inhaled beta-agonist therapy is complex. If patients present with acute severe asthma to an emergency department without having taken bronchodilator therapy previously, then additional bronchodilation would be likely with the addition of anticholinergic therapy to even relatively high doses of beta-agonist therapy. Conversely, those who present to an emergency department with severe asthma and who have already employed large doses of inhaled beta-agonist therapy are unlikely to experience much benefit from the addition of ipratropium bromide, nor are they likely to respond much to higher doses of beta-agonists.

Studies on acute asthma are performed in carefully supervised settings, usually within the emergency department, and are not necessarily generalizable. Therefore care is required when applying the results to asthma management within the community. For example, 24% of patients had been treated with nebulized bronchodilator prior to emergency department attendance in the New Zealand study, and the prior use of nebulized beta-agonists and higher serum salbutamol levels were both associated with more severe asthma on presentation. Whether this simply reflects the severity of the attack, is a consequence of an adverse effect of employing high doses of inhaled beta-agonist therapy (e.g., tachyphylaxis), or is a consequence of an indirect mechanism (i.e., delay in seeking medical attention), is impossible to say. However, the 8% of patients who had taken anticholinergic therapy during the acute attack did not present with more severe asthma, and prior inhaled anticholinergic therapy did not affect response to subsequent therapy. While concern persists about the potential adverse effect of overusing short-acting inhaled beta-agonists in high doses in unsupervised settings (33), an argument could be mounted that smaller doses of beta-agonist therapy be used in the community augmented with the very safe but less efficacious ipratropium bromide.

V. Does Ipratropium Bromide Contribute to Improvements in Clinical Outcomes?

Most studies that have evaluated the place of ipratropium bromide in acute asthma have employed one to three doses and used change in lung function as the primary outcome measurement. To address the question of whether ipratropium bromide contributes to an improvement in clinical outcome would require multiple dosing studies performed over many hours. Brophy et al. (34) assessed the question of optimum length of therapy with nebulized ipratropium in 106 patients admitted with acute asthma. All patients received 60 hours of nebulized salbutamol at 6-hour intervals and received systemic corticosteroids and theophylline as necessary. During the initial 12 hours all patients received nebulized ipratropium. They were then randomized into one of three groups: ipratropium for 36 hours, then placebo; ipratropium for 60 hours; or placebo. There was no difference in FEV_1 among the three groups at study end, but both groups who received additional ipratropium were discharged earlier than those who received ipratropium for 12 hours only ($P = .02$). It is hard to imagine, however, how the type of inhaled therapy might contribute to reducing the length of hospitalization when used in association with other management including oral steroid therapy.

One might realistically expect only short-term benefits from the addition of ipratropium bromide to beta-agonist therapy. Schuh et al. (35) showed both better bronchodilatation and reduced hospitalization with the addition of ipratopium to beta-agonist in their emergency department study on children with acute severe asthma. In their study, all patients received nebulized salbutamol 0.15 mg/kg per dose for three doses over 60 min. In addition they were randomized into one of three groups: (1) those who received ipratropium bromide 250 µg with each dose of salbutamol; (2) those who received one dose of 250 µg of ipratropium bromide with the first dose of nebulized salbutamol; and (3) those who received no ipratropium bromide. After 100 min, the mean percentage of predicted improvement for group 1 was 23.3%, for group 2 18.1%, and for group 3 13% ($P = .001$). The differences were even larger in those children with a baseline FEV_1 of <29% of predicted, who also exhibited a significant reduction in the need for hospitalization ($P = .03$).

In Lanes' combined analysis (26) of three recently completed emergency department studies in adult asthma, worse clinical outcomes were noted in the salbutamol group than in the group who had ipratropium added. The pooled analysis of 1064 patients revealed an 8% lower risk of need for additional emergency department treatment after administration of ipratropium bromide (RR = 0.92, 95% Cl = 0.84, 1) compared with salbutamol alone. Further, the risk of hospital admission for asthma during the 24 hours after initial treatment was 17% in the group receiving beta-agonist therapy only and 14% in the group receiving combination therapy (RR = 0.83, 95% Cl = 0.69, 1.1). Such improvements in clinical outcome, though small, appear similar in size to the improvements observed in lung function. While McFadden et al. (36)

concluded there was no benefit from adding ipratropium to standard beta-agonist therapy in the emergency department management of acute asthma, they found a small, nonsignificant improvement in lung function (4.3% predicted PEFR [$P = .11$]) and reduction in admission rate (25% vs. 28% [$P = .3$]) in the group receiving ipratropium. Although patients were not randomized in their study, and although they utilized a relatively crude lung function outcome (PEFR, with levels <100 L/min accepted as zero, and with no quality assurance program) and committed a type II error (n = 254), the results are not too dissimilar to the three larger studies on acute asthma in adults (23–25). In all four studies there are small improvements in clinical outcome which seem to mirror the small improvements in lung function.

VI. Is There a Pharmacoeconomic Argument for the Use of Inhaled Ipratropium Bromide in Acute Asthma?

No study has specifically addressed this question though it is of critical importance. In the New Zealand study (23), which was undertaken to evaluate the place of combination therapy in the management of acute asthma, there were fewer admissions in the combined ipratropium and salbutamol group (15.3%) than in the salbutamol-alone group (22.3%). These results were similar to those of the Canadian study (25), where patients in the salbutamol group (11.2%) were more likely to be admitted to the hospital than those receiving combination therapy (5.9%). When the cost of nebulized ipratropium is considered, the net benefit from adding ipratropium bromide to salbutamol 2.5 mg in New Zealand for the 330 patients recruited into the study was $NZ12,500 (unpublished observation) (conversion rate NZ$ to $US 0.65 approx), and would be substantially higher in countries where the cost of hospitalization is greater (e.g., United States and Canada). While the question remains whether similar benefits would have been seen if higher doses of beta-agonist were employed, if the results of this study were extrapolated to the whole of the New Zealand emergency department population of asthmatics, this would translate to an annual saving of $NZ118,000 (New Zealand population, 3.6 million).

VII. Are There Patient Subgroups Who Derive Particular Benefit from Anticholinergic Therapy?

It has been postulated that patients who have a fixed component of airways obstruction are more likely to have a significant vagal component to airway narrowing and therefore to benefit from anticholinergic therapy. However, none of the studies performed on ipratropium bromide show significant benefit for patients who are elderly (and who are more likely to have an element of fixed obstruction). In the New Zealand and Canadian studies (23,25), patients who were older were less likely to derive benefit from any form of nebulised bronchodilator therapy.

Patients who stated that their asthma attack was triggered as a result of a viral infection were more likely to derive benefit from the addition of anticholinergic therapy in all three studies reviewed by Lanes et al. (26). The improvement in FEV_1 for those who considered they had suffered an URTI was 105 mL greater for those randomized to ipratropium ($P = .02$), whereas no benefit was seen in those who did not have an URTI when ipratropium was added ($P = .72$). Given that there was no effort made to ascertain whether a virus was incriminated as the cause of the asthma attack, the association between attacks induced by viruses and benefit from ipratropium may in fact be even greater. Since viruses can contribute to an increase in bronchial hyperresponsiveness by increasing cholinergic responsiveness (37), an explanation for this observation exists, though clearly more research is required. Since children (38) are more likely than adults (39) to suffer acute exacerbations of asthma as a consequence of a viral illness, the association could also explain why it appears easier to show a benefit from the addition of ipratropium to beta-agonists in acute asthma management in children (34,35,40–43) than in adults. (Children are also more likely to access emergency departments with less severe asthma and to have consumed less bronchodilator therapy than adults prior to attendance, which may explain why children appear more responsive to bronchodilator therapy including ipratropium (44), since age per se does not influence bronchodilator response (45).)

Four studies (16,21,35,46) have shown that patients with the most severe asthma on presentation to the emergency department ($FEV_1 < 1$ L, PEF <140 L/min) do better with the addition of ipratropium bromide to beta-agonist therapy. Undoubtedly these results have influenced international guideline development on acute asthma management since it is suggested that ipratropium be reserved as second-line therapy and in patients with severe asthma who are not responding to beta-agonist therapy (1–3). However, three studies (22,23,25) have shown that patients with the most severe asthma ($FEV_1 < 1$ L, PEF < 60 L/min) derive less benefit. These differences may best be explained by differences in study design. In two of the four studies (16,21) showing a positive relationship between severity of asthma on presentation and response to ipratropium, patients were excluded if they had been administered nebulized beta-agonist therapy within 6 hours of ED attendance. However, prior nebulized beta-agonist therapy did not exclude patients recruited into any of the three studies showing a negative correlation. Further, in our study (23), 28% of patients had been administered a nebulizer prior to attendance; these patients not only had more severe asthma on attendance, but also responded less well to any bronchodilator therapy, including ipratropium.

VIII. Summary

The addition of anticholinergic therapy to standard beta-agonist nebulized therapy confers a small improvement in lung function and translates into a small clinical benefit. Whether this advantage is still observed when higher doses of beta-agonist therapy are employed, remains unclear. Carefully designed studies to evaluate this question using sufficient sample sizes, appropriate clinical outcome measurements, and pharmacoeconomic analysis are still required. Subgroups who seem to exhibit particular benefit from anticholinergic therapy are those who have consumed little previous bronchodilator therapy, those who have had an attack precipitated by a viral illness, and possibly children.

Because of its excellent safety profile a strong argument can be mounted for employing 0.5 mg ipratropium in association with 2.5 mg salbutamol rather than 5 mg salbutamol in managing asthma attacks in the community, where patients may be less carefully supervised than exists in the hospital setting. Other factors, such as the presence of troublesome coughing or a previously demonstrated response to ipratropium bromide, may also influence the clinician's prescribing habits.

References

1. British Thoracic Society. Guidelines for management of asthma. Thorax 1993; 48:S1–S24.
2. Asthma Management Handbook. Australia: National Asthma Campaign, 1996: 32–35.
3. Guidelines for the Diagnosis and Management of Asthma (EPR-2). NIH Publication No. 97-4051A, 1997.
4. Lin TY, Sauter D, Newman T, Shirleaf J, Walters J, Tavakol M. Continuous versus intermittent salbutamol nebulization in the treatment of acute asthma. Ann Emerg Med 1993; 22:1847–1853.
5. Rudnitsky GS, Eberlein RS, Schoffstall JM, Mazur JE, Spivey WH. Comparison

of intermittent and continuously nebulized salbutamol for treatment of asthma in an urban emergency department. Ann Emerg Med 1993; 22:1842–1846.
6. Seigel D, Sheppard D, Gelb A, et al. Aminophylline increases the toxicity but not the efficacy of an inhaled B-adrenergic agonist in the treatment of acute exacerbations of asthma. Am Rev Respir Dis 1985; 132:283–286.
7. Cheong B, Reynolds S, Rajan KG, Ward MJ. A comparison of intravenous with nebulised salbutamol in the treatment of acute severe asthma. Br Med J 1988; 297:448–450.
8. Lawford P, Jones BMJ, Milledge JS. Comparison of intravenous and nebulised salbutamol in initial treatment of severe asthma. Br Med J 1978; 1:84.
9. Williams SJ, Winner SJ, Clark TJH. Comparison of inhaled and intravenous terbutaline in acute severe asthma. Thorax 1981; 36:629–631.
10. Salmeron S, Brochard L, Mal H. Nebulized versus intavenous salbutamol in hypercapnic acute asthma: a multicenter, double-blind, randomized study. Am J Respir Crit Care Med 1994; 149:1466–1470.
11. Leahy B, Gomm SA, Allen SC. Comparison of nebulised salbutamol with nebulised ipratropium bromide in acute asthma. B J Dis Chest 1983; 82:1012–1018.
12. Watson WTA, Becker AB, Simons FER. Comparison of ipratropium solution, fenoterol solution, and their combination administered by nebulizer and face mask to children with acute asthma. J Allergy Clin Immunol 1988; 82:1012–1018.
13. Pierce RJ, Allen CJ, Campbell AH. A comparative study of atropine methonitrate salbutamol and their combination in airways obstruction. Thorax 1979; 34:45–50.
14. Gross NJ. Sch1000: a new anticholinergic bronchodilator. Am Rev Respir Dis 1975; 112:823–828.
15. Ward MJ, Fentem PH, Smith WHR, Davies D. Ipratropium bromide in acute asthma. Br Med J 1981; 282:598–600.
16. Rebuck AS, Chapman KR, Abboud R, Pare PD, Kreisman H, Wolkove N. Nebulized anticholinergic and sympathomimetic treatment of asthma and chronic obstructive airways disease in the emergency room. Am J Med 1987; 82:59–64.
17. Bryant D. Nebulised ipratropium bromide in the treatment of acute asthma. Chest 1988, 88:24–28.
18. Summers Q, Tarala RA. Nebulized ipratropium in the treatment of acute asthma. Chest 1990; 97:430–434.
19. Ward MJ. The role of anticholinergic drugs in acute asthma. In: Cross NJ, ed. Anticholinergic Therapy in Obstructive Airways Disease. London: Franklin Scientific Publications, 1993:155–162.
20. Higgins RM, Stradling JR, Lane DJ. Should ipratropium bromide be added to beta-agonist in the treatment of acute severe asthma? Chest 1988; 94:718–722.
21. O'Driscoll BR, Taylor RJ, Horsley MG, Chambers DK, Bernstein A. Nebulised salbutamol with and without ipratropium bromide in the treatment of acute severe asthma? Lancet 1989; 1:1418–1420.

22. Roeseler J, Reynaert MS. A comparison of fenoterol and fenoterol ipratropium nebulisation treatment in acute asthma. Acta Ther 1987; 13:571–576.
23. Garrett JE, Town Gl, Rodwell P, Kelly AM. Nebulized salbutamol with and without ipratropium bromide in the treatment of acute asthma. J Allergy Clin Immunol 1997; 100:165–170.
24. Karpel JP, Schector EN, Fanta C, et al. A comparison of ipratropium and salbutamol vs. salbutamol alone for the treatment of acute asthma. Chest 1996; 110: 611–616.
25. Fitzgerald JM, Grunfeld A, Pare PD, et al. The clinical efficacy of combination nebulized anticholinergic and adrenergic bronchodilators versus nebulized adrenergic bronchodilator alone in acute asthma. Chest 1997.
26. Lanes SF, Garrett JE, Wentworth CE, Fitzgerald JM, Karpel JP. The effect of adding ipratropium bromide to salbutamol in the treatment of acute asthma: a pooled analysis of three trials. Chest 1998. In press.
27. Enright PL, Johnson LR, Connett JE, Voelker H, Buist AS. Spirometry in the Lung Health Study 1. Methods and quality control. Am Rev Respir Dis 1991; 143:1215–1223.
28. Ward MJ, Macfarlane JT, Davies D. A place for ipratropium bromide in the treatment of severe acute asthma. B J Dis Chest 1985; 79:394–398.
29. Rossing TH, Fanta CH, McFadden ER. The effect of outpatient treatment of asthma with beta-agonists on the response to sympathomimetics in an emergency room. Am J Med 1983; 75:781–784.
30. Janson C, Boe J, Borman G, Mossberg B, Svedmyr N. Bronchodilator intake and plasma levels on admission for acute severe asthma. Eur Respir J 1992; 5: 80–85.
31. Boe J, Carisson LG, Hetta L, Karlson B, Ljungholm K. Acute asthma-plasma levels and effect of terbutaline IV injections. Eur Respir Dis 1985; 67: 261–268.
32. Garrett J, Frankel A, Lanes S, Rodwell P, Kelly AM, Town GI. Factors predicting severity and response to therapy in acute asthma. Am J Respir Crit Care Med 1995; 151:A380.
33. Spitzer WO, Suissa S, Ernst P, et al. The use of beta-agonists and the risk of death or near death from asthma. N Engl J Med 1992; 326:501–506.
34. Brophy C, Ahmed B, Bayston S, Arnold A, McGivern D, Greenstone M. How long should Atrovent be given in acute severe asthma? Am J Respir Care Med 1996; 153(4 pt 2):A351.
35. Schuh S, Johnson DW, Callahan S, Canny G, Levison H. Efficacy of frequent nebulized ipratropium bromide added to frequent high-dose salbutamol therapy in severe childhood asthma. J Pediatr 1995; 126:639–645.
36. McFadden ER, El Sanadi N, Strauss L, et al. The influence of parasympatholytics on the resolution of acute attacks of asthma. Am J Med. 1997; 102:7–13.
37. Corne JM, Holgate ST. Mechanisms of virus induced exacerbations of asthma. Thorax 1997; 52:380–389.
38. Johnston S, Pattemore P, Sanderson G, et al. Community study of the role of

viral infections in exacerbations of asthma in 9–11 year old children. BMJ 1995; 310:1225–1229.
39. Hudgel DW, Langston L, Selner J, McIntosh K. Viral and bacterial infections in adults with chronic asthma. Am Rev Respir Dis 1979; 120:393.
40. Quereshi F, Zaritsky A, Lakkis H. Efficacy of nebulised ipratropium bromide in severely asthmatic children. Ann Emerg Med 1997; 29:205–211.
41. Beck R, Robertson C, Galdes-Sebalt M, Levison H. Combined salbutamol and ipratropium bromide by inhalation in the treatment of severe acute asthma. J Pediatr 1985; 107:605–608.
42. Reisman J, Galdes-Sebalt M, Kazim F, Canny G, Levison H. Frequent administration by inhalation of salbutamol and ipratropium bromide in the initial management of severe acute asthma in children. J Allergy Clin Immunol 1988; 81: 16–20.
43. DeStefano G, Bonetti S, Bonizzato C, Valletta EA, Piacentini GL, Boner AL. Additive effect of salbutamol and ipratropium bromide in the treatment of bronchospasm in children. Ann Allergy 1990; 65:260–262.
44. Garrett J, Mulder J, Wong-Toi H. Characteristics of asthmatics using an urban accident and emergency department. NZ Med J 1988; 101:359–361.
45. Kradjan WA, Driesner NK, Abuan TH, Emmick G, Schoene RB. Effect of age on bronchodilator response. Chest 1992; 101:1545–1551.
46. Rossing TH, Fanta C, McFadden ER. A controlled trial of the use of a single versus combined drug therapy in the treatment of acute episodes of asthma. Am Rev Respir Dis 1981; 123:190–194.

5
Use of Anticholinergics in Perennial Rhinitis

ALBERT F. FINN, JR.

Medical University of South Carolina
Charleston, South Carolina

I. Introduction

Rhinitis is a common disease affecting millions of people worldwide. In England, epidemiologic studies from the 1980s have shown the prevalence to be approximately 25% in adults (1). In the United States, a recent study assessing the socioeconomic impact of rhinitis estimated that in 1987, 39 million individuals in the United States had allergic rhinitis with approximately 12 million being pediatric patients. Furthermore, the research indicated that in 1994 dollars the direct and indirect costs would be approximately $1.25 billion to care for this 1987 cohort.

These data were derived from a national medical expenditure survey of approximately 14,000 U.S. households (2). Data derived from a national health interview survey in 1994 resulted in the estimate that 10% of the U.S. population (approximately 26 million individuals) had allergic rhinitis (3). However, the lower prevalence of rhinitis among the population likely reflects an inability to include all individuals who had rhinitis as characterized by the prototypical symptoms of nasal congestion, rhinorrhea, and nasal pruritus or sneezing. A 1993 study utilizing the National Family Opinion questionnaire found an approximate prevalence of allergic rhinitis of 14.2% (35.9 million) based on self-reporting by the individuals. However, the study also revealed that if the prevalence of nasal or ocular symptoms consistent with rhinitis was used as diagnostic criteria, the prevalence may be as high as 31.5% (4).

Using the economic data derived from the same self-administered questionnaire, an evaluation of costs related to the care of allergic rhinitis in the United States was performed. This evaluation resulted in an estimate of costs of $3.4 billion to treat allergic rhinitis in the United States in 1993 (5). Regardless of the methodology or region of the world, one-quarter or more of the world's population suffers from rhinitis, and the costs for the care of rhinitis are significant. The importance of rhinitis around the globe has prompted international efforts to define rhinitis, its causes, and approaches to treatment (6).

The symptom complexes typically associated with rhinitis are commonly found in the population. The causes for these symptoms are derived from various pathogenic mechanisms. Generally, the mechanisms are divided between allergic and nonallergic classifications. Allergic rhinitis results from mechanisms that require a specific IgE-mediated process, with subsequent inflammation of mucosal surfaces. Inhalant allergens that result in inflammation of the nasal airways are divided into seasonal and perennial types. Seasonal allergens arise from botanical species that pollinate during a defined growing period each year. Examples of seasonal allergens include pollens from grasses, trees, and weeds. Perennial allergic rhinitis is dependent upon the allergen being present throughout the year. Generally, these allergens arise from dust mites, cockroaches, fungi, and pets. Their respective allergens originate from various structural components and are generally in the environment throughout the year. Dust mite allergens as well as pet and cockroach allergens are common within the home and have been documented to be directly responsible for rhinitic symptoms (7–9). Community-based studies, such as one performed in London, found that of the 25% of adults with rhinitis, approximately 20% had perennial symptoms, and of these, 50% to 68% were allergic by skin testing (1).

Once allergic mechanisms are excluded as the cause for perennial rhinitis, the remaining individuals are generally deemed to have perennial nonallergic rhinitis. These individuals, who represent up to 5% of the adult population, have rhinitic symptoms in the absence of demonstrable IgE-mediated hypersensitivity (10,11). Furthermore, the presence or absence of eosinophilia found on cytologic examination of nasal airway smears allows further subcategorization to nonallergic rhinitis with or without eosinophilia (12).

The general therapeutic approach to rhinitis is aimed at both symptomatic relief and interference with pathophysiologic mechanisms. Perennial nonallergic rhinitis, in the absence of infectious or systemic disease, is treated symptomatically. Hence, agents used to treat perennial nonallergic rhinitis are directed at attenuating the symptoms of nasal congestion and excessive rhinorrhea. Sneezing and nasal pruritus tend to be less common in these patients. Symptomatic relief is generally obtained by the use of systemic and topical decongestants, topical nasal corticosteroids, and topical anticholinergic agents. In perennial allergic rhinitis, treatment generally includes avoidance of the allergens responsible for the nasal airway inflammation, use of pharmacotherapeutic agents capable of attenuating the allergic inflammation, and medications for symptomatic relief and immunotherapy. Symptomatic relief is achieved through the use of decongestants, anticholinergics, and antihistamines. Systemic and topical nasal corticosteroids are used for attenuating the allergic inflammation, and immunotherapy is directed at immunomodulating the IgE-mediated process.

The focus of this chapter is to explore the use of anticholinergics in the treatment of a common and costly health care problem, namely, perennial nonallergic and allergic rhinitis. Anticholinergics are pharmacologic agents that directly address the glandular hypersecretion identified in both perennial allergic and nonallergic rhinitis. Their topical use has been found to be efficacious in the treatment of perennial allergic and nonallergic rhinitis in both pediatric and adult patients.

II. Pathophysiology of Perennial Rhinitis

The symptoms of nasal congestion, glandular hypersecretion, and sneezing or nasal pruritus are the prototypical symptoms of rhinitis. In allergic rhinitis, these symptoms arise from pathophysiologic mechanisms localized in the upper respiratory tract (7,13). Airborne allergens are respired into the nasal airways and make physical contact with the nasal mucosa. Upon contact, the respective allergens derived from particles such as animal dander, dust mite fecal pellets, and fungal spores gain access to mast cells within the mucosal surface. Degranulation of the mast cells initially results in the immediate release of preformed mediators such as histamine, heparin, and tryptase; leukotrienes (LTC4, LTD4, and LTE4) and prostaglandin D_2 are elaborated subsequently from arachidonic acid. Histamine that is released during the early allergic reaction results in increased vascular permeability of the postcapillary venule, leading to vascular leak and mucosal edema. Additionally, the plasma transudate contributes to secretions localizing in the nasal airways. Constriction of draining vessels from vascular sinusoids within the nasal mucosa results in engorgement of the vascular sinusoids in the mucosal tissue and in decreased patency of the nasal airways.

C-fibers that are nonadrenergic, noncholinergic afferent sensory neurons have histamine receptors. They facilitate centrally mediated reflexes, which results in sneezing and glandular secretion. The glandular secretion occurs via parasympathetic efferents to submucosal serous and mucous glands. Release of acetylcholine stimulates M_1 and M_3 receptors found in the lamina propria, resulting in glandular exocytosis. This parasympathetic mediated reflex is responsible for the contribution of glandular products to nasal secretions. Summarily, nasal airway secretions are a composite of glandular secretions and plasma transudate (14–22).

The late-phase reaction, which characteristically occurs 6 to 8 hours after contact with allergens, is heralded by the influx of eosinophils and lymphocytes. Activated eosinophils release various mediators, including eosinophilic cationic protein and major basic protein. Lymphocytes infiltrating into the area are primarily of the CD4 phenotype, which can elaborate interleukin-5, thereby sustaining the eosinophilic population. Infiltrating lymphocytes elaborate many cytokines, including interleukin-3, granulocyte macrophage colony-stimulating factor, connective tissue-activating peptide III, and others that are known to be histamine-releasing factors for basophils and mast cells. Continued degranulation of mast cells and basophils results in persistent secretion of histamine and other mediators during the late-phase component of the IgE-mediated inflammation (9,13).

Perennial nonallergic rhinitis is a diagnosis of exclusion. Patients who report characteristic symptoms of nasal airway obstruction, rhinorrhea, and nasal pruritus or sneezing in the absence of demonstrable allergic disease are included in this designation. Other possible etiologies for nonallergic rhinitis include rhinitis medicamentosa, coexistent thyroid disease or pregnancy, atrophic rhinitis, sinonasal polyposis, and upper-airway malignancies. Patients with perennial nonallergic rhinitis complain of nasal obstruction, excessive nasal secretions, and, less commonly, sneezing or nasal pruritus. Perennial nonallergic rhinitis can be subcategorized further into perennial nonallergic rhinitis with and without eosinophilia (1). This depends on the presence of abundant eosinophils on cytologic examination of the nasal mucosa (12).

III. Cholinergic Mechanisms in Perennial Rhinitis

Anterior rhinorrhea and postnasal drainage are symptoms described commonly by patients with rhinitis (10). These symptoms result from glandular hypersecretion and generalized mucorrhea of the nasal airway. The nasal mucosa of the upper airway is innervated peripherally by the parasympathetic nerve fibers of the autonomic nervous system. Parasympathetic fibers, found running with motor fibers of the seventh cranial nerve, synapse in the sphenopalatine ganglia. They pass through the Vidian canal and proceed to the nasal mucosa. Acetylcholine, as well as neurogenic peptides such as vasoactive intestinal peptide (VIP), is released from these postganglionic neurons. These parasympathetic fibers result in glandular hypersecretion from both goblet cells and submucosal seromucinous glands.

Additionally, glands can be stimulated by the local release of neuropeptides from the nociceptive C-fibers. The nociceptive C-fibers form the afferent arm for central reflexes in the nose which traverse with the first and second divisions of the trigeminal nerve. Mediators that elicit sensory nerve stimulation with activation of central nerve reflexes include histamine, bradykinin, and serotonin (10). Moreover, capsaicin stimulates the nociceptive sensory nerves and causes cholinergic-mediated hypersecretion via the same parasympathetic nerves that are responsible for the reflex hypersecretion following histamine activation of nociceptive C-fibers (14). These parasympathetic efferents arise from the superior salivatory nucleus of the brainstem. It is noteworthy that individuals with atopy and nonallergic rhinitis have evidence of glandular hyperactivity when challenged with either histamine or methacholine (23–26).

Five types of muscarinic receptors have been identified (M_1 to M_5). Within the mucosal surface of the nose, receptors subtypes M_1 and M_3 have been localized (27). The M_1-receptor subtype results in secretion from mucous and serous glands. The M_3 receptor subtype has been localized to mucous and serous glands as well as blood vessels. One function of the M_3 receptor is considered to be secretion of glandular products. In addition, nasal congestion mediated by vasodilation may be a result of acetylcholine at the M_3 receptor or secondary to vasoactive intestinal peptide that is colocalized in the parasympathetic nerve terminals (14). M_2 subtype receptors which have been localized in the human lung are believed to regulate the parasympathetic response via negative feedback. However, they have not been detected in the nasal mucosa. The M_1 and M_3 muscarinic receptors found in the nasal mucosa are stimulated via acetylcholine or methacholine. Cholinergic antagonists, including atropine (Fig. 1) and ipratropium bromide, are capable of blocking these receptors

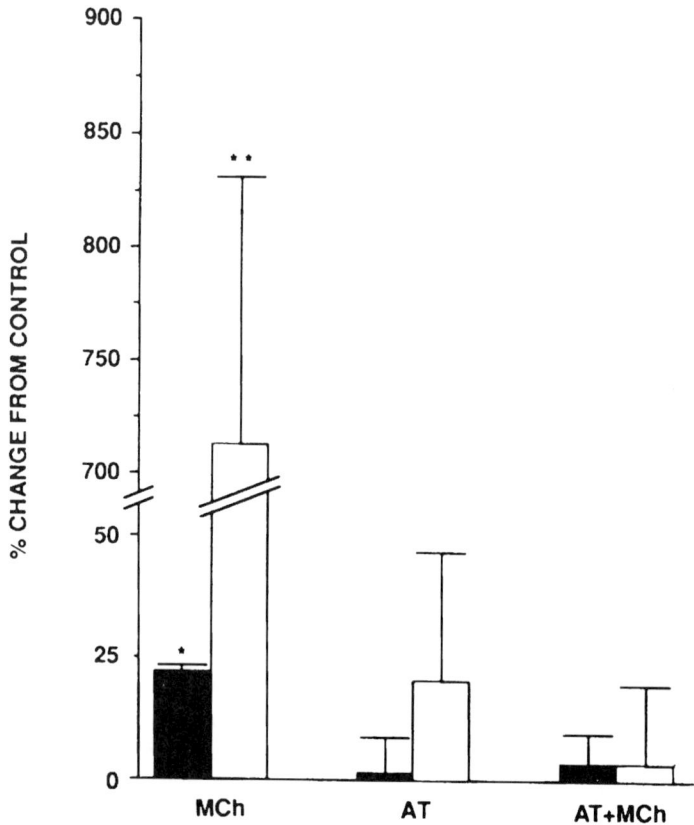

Figure 1 Inhibitory effect of atropine (AT) on methacholine (MCh)-induced secretions in vitro. Stimulation of human turbinate explants with methacholine results in production of respiratory glycoconjugate from submucosal mucous glands (solid bars) and lactoferrin from submucosal serous glands (open bars). Atropine results in significant suppression of glandular secretions. Methacholine versus atropine plus methacholine data were compared by paired Student's t-test (mean + SEM; n= 6). **$P < .01$; *$P < .05$. (From Ref. 15.)

(15,28–31). These cholinergic receptors and their effects are responsible for the glandular hypersecretion seen in antigen challenge and cold, dry air challenge models (32).

IV. Anticholinergic Agents in Perennial and Nonallergic Rhinitis

With the understanding that glandular secretions of the nasal airway are elicited by parasympathetic mechanisms, anticholinergic agents that block the peripheral muscarinic receptors in the nasal mucosa were investigated for their efficacy in rhinitis (28–32). The first agent to be studied as therapeutic was atropine methonitrate. Protocols used direct provocation with agents such as methacholine, histamine, antigens, and cold, dry air. These studies revealed significant attenuation of the rhinorrhea by utilizing atropine in individuals with perennial allergic rhinitis as well as in individuals with gustatory rhinitis and cold, dry air–induced rhinorrhea (33,34). However, atropine is absorbed systemically and does result in systemic anticholinergic side effects. These side effects include dryness of the mouth, somnolence, and urinary retention.

Quaternary ammonium muscarinic receptor antagonists are unable to cross the blood-brain barrier. With this in mind, pharmaceutical development of ipratropium bromide (Fig. 2) resulted in an anticholinergic agent that had limited systemic absorption. Ipratropium bromide is a quaternary amine, and its cationic molecule is not absorbed across physiologic membranes to any significant degree (31). Thus, absorption of ipratropium bromide from the respiratory tract or gastrointestinal tract is diminutive. This unappreciable degree of systemic absorption and its limited egress across the blood-brain barrier due to its cationic structure result in negligible central nervous system side

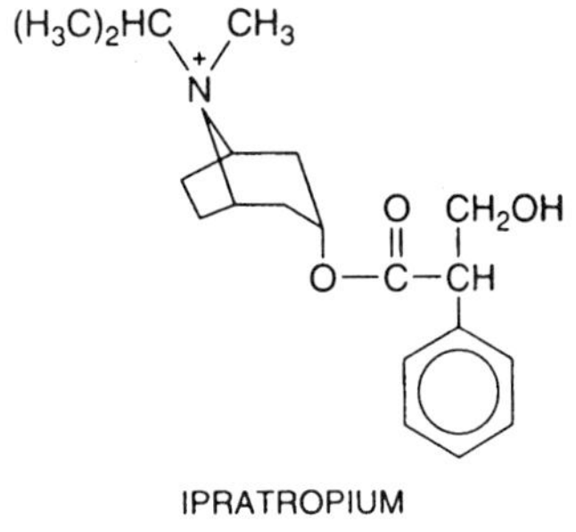

Figure 2 Chemical structure of ipratroprium bromide.

effects. Ipratropium bromide has been formulated for intranasal application, using a chlorofluorocarbon delivery in Europe and using an aqueous-based formulation in the United States.

The formulation of intranasal ipratropium bromide, which is delivered using chlorofluorocarbons, has been intensively investigated in several thousand patients. Studies have utilized dosages ranging from 20 to 640 μg per day. These investigations have revealed the formulation to be safe and effective in the control of rhinorrhea associated with perennial nonallergic rhinitis. The chlorofluorocarbon-based ipratropium bromide device (ATROVENT MDI) delivers 20 μg of ipratropium bromide monohydrate. The recommended dosage is two actuations (40 μg per nostril) two to three times daily. Side effects that have been recorded with this preparation include dryness and irritation of the nasal mucosa, epistaxis, and nasal airway congestion. The side effects noted are, in part, related to the use of chlorofluorocarbon in this preparation. As such, this preparation has limited utility in clinical disease for perennial nonallergic rhinitis (35). However, chlorofluorocarbon-based ipratropium bromide had no demonstrable effect on olfaction, ciliary function, or air-conditioning capacity of the nose (36,37).

An aqueous-based formulation of ipratropium bromide avowed exiguous side effects and cogent results. Initial studies utilizing ipratropium nasal spray in a 0.03% concentration revealed significant improvement in symptoms within the first day of therapy and a maximal benefit within 2 weeks of treatment (35). The 0.03% aqueous-based formulation did not result in significant or severe side effects. Adverse events with aqueous intranasal ipratropium bromide 0.03%, when compared to saline vehicle, were as follows: transient episodes of epistaxis—9% versus 5%; nasal dryness—5% versus 1%. The dosage used was two sprays of 0.03% aqueous-based ipratropium bromide (42 μg) two to three times daily.

Following discontinuation of the preparation, no rebound of symptoms occurred with other agents (38). Hence, the use of intranasal ipratropium bromide as an anticholinergic agent is generally safe.

Studies involving allergic and nonallergic perennial rhinitis patients reveal the efficacy of topical intranasal ipratropium bromide in a concentration of 0.03%. Two groups of patients with allergic perennial rhinitis were studied for periods of 4 and 8 weeks, respectively (38). During each of these trials, efficacy was demonstrated in improving the severity and in limiting the duration of the rhinorrhea. Three additional studies were performed in individuals who had perennial nonallergic rhinitis, again for periods of 4 and 8 weeks. Each of the three studies resulted in the findings of a decrease in the severity and in the duration of the rhinorrhea compared to the placebo (39–41). Notably, the placebo used was the vehicle without the active drug. Furthermore, quality-of-life issues were addressed in selected studies assessing the efficacy of the nasal ipratropium bromide, and the participants' moods and physical activity also improved (40,41).

Finally, extended use of intranasal ipratropium bromide 0.03% yielded findings of improvement of rhinorrhea, as assessed by both the study participants and the study evaluators (42). The extended trials did not reveal any adverse events related to extended use. In addition, during this period the use of intranasal ipratropium bromide did not increase adverse events when used in combination with antihistamines, decongestants, or nasal steroids.

As discussed earlier in the chapter, rhinitis is typified by symptoms including rhinorrhea, congestion, and nasal pruritus or sneezing. While the use of topical anticholinergic agents ameliorates the primary symptom of rhinorrhea, minimal benefit is afforded to nasal congestion, nasal pruritus, or sneezing. Therefore, topical anticholinergics may be used in combination with other therapeutic agents used for rhinitis.

Two studies specifically investigated the combination of topical intranasal ipratropium bromide with systemic antihistamines and topical intranasal corticosteroids. Intranasal ipratropium bromide 0.03% at a dosing regimen of two sprays each nostril TID (42 µg per nostril) plus terfenadine 60 mg BID is significantly more effective than the vehicle combined with terfenadine in reducing the severity and duration of rhinorrhea from baseline (43). Further, the combination of intranasal ipratropium bromide nasal spray 0.03% administered two sprays per nostril (42 µg) TID with intranasal beclomethasone effected a 10% to 15% improved reduction in the rhinorrhea versus intranasal ipratropium bromide or intranasal beclomethasone alone in both allergic and nonallergic perennial rhinitis (44). The combination of intranasal ipratropium bromide with systemic terfenadine and intranasal beclomethasone was not associated with any higher incidence of adverse reactions over the individual agents alone (43,44). The most recent investigation involving intranasal ipratropium bromide focused on its use in the pediatric population. Intranasal ipratropium bromide was studied for its efficacy in both perennial allergic and nonallergic rhinitis in participants 6 to 18 years of age. The use of ipratropium nasal spray 0.03% two sprays each nostril (42 µg) over a 1-month period manifested no adverse outcomes. The study revealed the drug to be effective in controlling rhinorrhea (45). An extension of this protocol over 6 months revealed equal safety and efficacy in controlling glandular hypersecretion as intranasal beclomethasone (46).

V. Summary

Parasympathetic efferents to the nasal mucosa synapse with their receptors found on submucosal seromucinous glands. These end organs can be stimulated to secrete glandular products via muscarinic receptors. Activation of glandular exocytosis can be precipitated by stimulation of nociceptive C-fibers with histamine or thermomechanical insult. Once activated, these sensory fibers serve as the afferent loop for the centrally mediated response of glandular secretion of the submucosal serous and mucous glands.

Glandular hypersecretion in the nasal airways occurs in the clinical diseases of perennial allergic and nonallergic rhinitis. Patients' described symptoms include anterior rhinorrhea and postnasal drainage.

Pharmacotherapeutic agents that can block the muscarinic receptors are capable of attenuating the mucorrhea and relieving symptoms. Atropine and other structurally related agents have limited clinical use because of systemic side effects. Quaternary ammonium compounds, such as ipratropium bromide, can be applied topically and have limited systemic absorption or toxicity. Currently, ipratropium bromide is the only quaternary ammonium compound available for clinical use. It has been found to be safe and effective in clinical disease states with excessive rhinorrhea. Extensive clinical investigations demonstrate its utility in the glandular hypersecretion associated with perennial allergic and nonallergic rhinitis.

References

1. Sibbald B, Rink E. Epidemiology of seasonal and perennial rhinitis. Clinical presentation and medical history. Thorax 1991; 46:895–901.
2. Malone DC, Lawson KA, Smith DH, Arrighi HM, Battista C. A cost of illness study of allergic rhinitis in the United States. J Allergy Clin Immunol 1997; 99: 22–27.
3. Adams PF, Marano MA. Current estimates from the National Health Interview Survey, 1994. Vital and Health Statistics. U.S. Dept of Health and Human Services publication (PHS) 96-1521. Series 10: No. 193. Hyattsville, MD: National Centers for Health Statistics, 1995.
4. Nathan RA, Meltzer EO, Selner JC, Storms W. Prevalence of allergic rhinitis in the United States. J Allergy Clin Immunol 1997; 99:S808–S814.
5. Storms W, Meltzer EO, Nathan RA, Selner JC. The economic impact of allergic rhinitis. J Allergy Clin Immunol 1997; 99:S820–S824.
6. International Rhinitis Management Working Group. International consensus report on the diagnosis and management of allergic rhinitis. Allergy 1994; 49:5–34.

7. Naclerio RM. Allergic rhinitis. N Engl J Med 1991; 325:860–868.
8. Meltzer EO, Schatz M, Zeiger RS. Allergic and nonallergic rhinitis. In: Middleton E Jr, Reed CE, Ellis EF, Adkinson NF, Yuninger JW, eds. Allergy: Principles and Practices. St. Louis: C.V. Mosby, 1988:1253–1289.
9. Rajakulasingam K, Anderson DF, Holgafe ST. Allergic rhinitis, nonallergic rhinitis, and ocular allergy. In: Kaplan AP, ed. Allergy. Philadelphia: W.B. Saunders, 1997:421–448.
10. Mygind N, Angyard A, Druce HM. Definition, classification, and terminology. In: Mygind N, Week B, eds. Allergic and vasomotor rhinitis; clinical aspects. Copenhagen: Munksgaard, 1985:15–20.
11. Mullarkey MF, Hill JS, Webb DR. Allergic and nonallergic rhinitis: their characterization with attention to the meaning of eosinophilia. J Allergy Clin Immunol 1980; 65:122–126.
12. Meltzer EO, Jalowayski AA. Nasal cytology in clinical practice. Am J Rhinol 1988; 2:47–54.
13. Baraniuk JN. Pathogenesis of allergic rhinitis. J Allergy Clin Immunol 1997; 99: S763–S772.
14. Baraniuk JN. Neural control of human nasal secretion. Pulm Pharmacol 1991; 4:1–12.
15. Mullol J, Raphael GD, Lundgren JD, et al. Comparison of human nasal mucosal secretion in vivo and in vitro. J Allergy Clin Immunol 1992; 89:584–592.
16. Shelhamer JH, Marom Z, Kaliner M. Immunologic and neuropharmacologic stimulation of mucous glycoprotein release from human airways in vitro. J Clin Invest 1980; 66:1400–1408.
17. Boat TF, Kleinerman JI. Human respiratory tract secretions. II. Effect of cholinergic and adrenergic agents on in vitro release of protein and mucous glycoprotein. Chest 1975; 67:32S–34S.
18. Paton CA, Shelhamer J, Marom Z, Logun C, Kaliner M. Analysis of human nasal mucous glycoproteins. Am J Otolaryngol 1984; 5:334–343.
19. Basbaum CB, Veki I, Brezina L, Nadel JA. Tracheal submucosal gland serous cells stimulated in vitro with adrenergic and cholinergic agonists: a morphometric study. Cell Tissue Res 1981; 220:481–498.
20. Raphael GD, Druce HM, Baraniuk JN, Kaliner MA. Pathophysiology of rhinitis. I. Assessment of the sources of protein in methacholine-induced nasal secretions. Am Rev Respir Dis 1988; 138:413–420.
21. Raphael GD, Meredith SD, Baraniuk JN, Druce HM, Banks SM, Kaliner MA. The pathophysiology of rhinitis. II. Assessment of the sources of protein in histamine-induced nasal secretions. Am Rev Respir Dis 1989; 139:791–800.
22. Raphael GD, Baraniuk JN, Kaliner MA. How and why the nose runs. J Allergy Clin Immunol 1991; 87:457–467.
23. Druce HM, Wright RH, Kossoff D, Kaliner MA. Cholinergic nasal hyperactivity in atopic subjects. J Allergy Clin Immunol 1985; 76:445–452.
24. Sjogren I, Jonsson L, Koling A, et al. The effect of ipratropium bromide on nasal

hypersecretion induced by methacholine in patients with vasomotor rhinitis. Acta Otolaryngol (Stockh) 1988; 106:453–459.
25. White MV. Nasal cholinergic hyperresponsiveness in atopic subjects studied out of season. J Allergy Clin Immunol 1993; 92:278–287.
26. Baroody FM, Wagenmann M, Naclerio RM. A comparison of the secretory response of the nasal mucosa to methacholine and histamine. J Appl Physiol 1993; 74:2661–2671.
27. White M. Muscarinic receptors in human airways. J Allergy Clin Immunol 1995; 95:1065–1068.
28. Dolorich J, Mukherjec J, Salvatori VA. Intranasal ipratropium bromide to control the hypersecretion of vasomotor rhinitis: a dose-response study. Am J Rhinol 1989; 3:221–224.
29. Baroody FM, Ford S, Lichtenstein LM, Kagey-Sobotka A, Naclerio RM. Physiologic responses and histamine release after nasal antigen challenge. Effect of atropine. Am J Respir Crit Care Med 1994; 149:1457–1465.
30. Jackson RT, Teichgraeber J. Low-dose topical atropine for rhinitis. Arch Otolaryngol 1981; 107:288–289.
31. Wood CC, Fireman P, Grossman J, Wecker M, MacGregor T. Product characteristics and pharmacokinetics of intranasal ipratropium bromide. J Allergy Clin Immunol 1995; 95(5 part 2):1111–1116.
32. Janowski R, Philip G, Togias A, Nacleno R. Demonstration of bilateral cholinergic secretory response after unilateral nasal cold, dry air challenge. Rhinology 1993; 31:97–100.
33. Raphael G, Hauptschein-Raphael M, Kaliner M. Gustatory rhinitis: a syndrome of food-induced rhinorrhea. J Allergy Clin Immunol 1989; 83:110–115.
34. Silvers W. The skier's nose. A model of cold-induced rhinorrhea. Ann Allergy 1991; 67:32–36.
35. Meltzer EO. Intranasal anticholinergic therapy of rhinorrhea. J Allergy Clin Immmunol 1992; 90(6):1055–1070.
36. Ohi M, Sakura Y, Murai S, Miyoshi Y. Effect of ipratropium bromide on nasal mucociliary transport. Rhinology 1984; 22:241–246.
37. Kumlien J, Drettner B. The effect of ipratropium bromide on the air conditioning capacity of the nose. Clin Otolaryngol 1985; 10:165–168.
38. Meltzer E, Orgel A, Bronsky E, et al. Ipratropium bromide aqueous nasal spray for patients with perennial allergic rhinitis: a study of its effect on their symptoms, quality of life, and nasal cytology. J Allergy Clin Immunol 1992; 90(2): 242–249.
39. Druce HM, Spector SL, Fireman P, et al. Double-blind study of intranasal ipratropium bromide in nonallergic perennial rhinitis. Ann Allergy 1992; 69:53–60.
40. Bronsky EA, Druce H, Findlay SR, et al. A clinical trial of ipratropium bromide nasal spray in patients with perennial rhinitis. J Allergy Clin Immunol 1995; 95(5 part 2):1117–1122.
41. Georgitis JW, Banov C, Boggs PB, et al. Ipratropium bromide nasal spray in

nonallergic rhinitis: efficacy, nasal cytological response, and patient evaluation on quality of life. Clin Exp Allergy 1993; 24:1049–1055.

42. Grossman J, Banov C, Boggs P, et al. Use of ipratropium bromide nasal spray in chronic treatment of nonallergic perennial rhinitis, alone and in combination with other perennial rhinitis medications. J Allergy Clin Immunol 1995; 95(5 part 2):1123–1127.

43. Finn A, Korenblatt P, Lumry W, et al. A randomized, double-blind comparison of combined use of ATROVENT nasal spray 0.03% (A) plus Seldane (S) versus S plus vehicle (V) in patients with allergic and nonallergic perennial rhinitis (APR and NAPR). Am J Respir Crit Care Med 1996; 153(4):A525.

44. Dockhorn R, Bronsky E, Chervinsky P, et al. A randomized, double-blind, six-week, placebo-controlled (V), parallel comparison of ATROVENT nasal spray 0.03% (A) alone, Beconase AQ (B) alone, and the combined use of A with B in patients with allergic and nonallergic perennial rhinitis (APR and NAPR). Am J Respir Crit Care Med 1996; 153(4):A525.

45. Meltzer EO, Orgel HA, Biondi R, et al. Ipratropium nasal spray in children with perennial rhinitis. Ann Allergy Asthma Immunol 1997; 78:485–491.

46. Milgrom H, Biondi R, Georgitis J, et al. Comparison of ipratropium bromide with beclomethasone diproprionate in the treatment of perennial rhinitis in children. Ann Allergy Asthma Immunol 1997; 78:125.

6

Pathogenesis and Treatment of Upper Respiratory Infections

SHELDON L. SPECTOR

University of California, Los Angeles, School of Medicine
Los Angeles, California

I. Introduction

The "common cold" has been called various names in the literature, including acute coryza, infectious rhinitis, acute nasal catarrh, acute nasal pharyngitis, or a viral upper respiratory infection (URI).

The average preschool child has six to 10 URIs per year. The average adult has approximately half that number or less, depending on variables such as exposure to the general public or to children, in particular (1). Interestingly, one-third of individuals who have a confirmed infection have no apparent cold symptoms.

Earlier statistics suggest that viral upper respiratory infections account for nearly 50% of all illnesses, and nearly 75% of illnesses in young infants (2,3). In 1992, the U.S. Department of Health and Human Services estimated that our total healthcare expenditures were in the neighborhood of $800 billion (4).

Thus, URIs of a viral nature are a leading cause of acute morbidity and have significant associated costs. Although URIs are mild, self-limited, and of short duration, they are a primary reason for industrial and school absenteeism (5–7). Each year, URIs account for 170 million days of restricted activity, 23 million days of school absence, and 25 million days of absence from work (7).

There are significant direct and indirect costs related to URIs. Direct costs include office visits including laboratory evaluations, as well as treatment. Americans spend from $1 million to $2 billion annually on the more than 800 over-the-counter cough and cold preparations available to them (8,9).

A portion of the direct cost for treatment of URIs is for inappropriate or ineffective medications. It has been estimated that unnecessary medications account for nearly 60% of the total prescription cost (10). Many cold preparations, such as decongestants/antihistamines or cough suppressants, have limited if any beneficial effect on the prominent symptom of rhinorrhea (11). Because of the viral etiology of URIs, antibiotics are not indicated treatment (5). Recent studies in the United States showed that 60% of cases of acute nasopharyngitis (e.g., common cold) were treated with antibiotics (12).

Even using the most conservative estimates of medication costs of $2.41 for a course of therapy (based on the Health Care Financing Administration wholesale cost of 250 mg of amoxicillin for 10 days) (13), this suggests that antibiotic use for URIs adds $35 million to the annual cost of care in the United States. It must be emphasized that this is a very conservative estimate, since data show that many of these office visits lead to the prescription of antibiotics more expensive than amoxicillin (12). In fact, in many cases, the antibiotics prescribed for URIs are more expensive than a typical physician's office visit.

Indirect costs for URIs include productivity losses related to lost workdays for adults who are sick and for adults who have to deal with sick children. Other indirect costs that are many times overlooked are those associated with lost opportunities to immunize young children. A large portion of children are not immunized on schedule, due to visits for URIs (14). This finding also suggests additional visits for immunizations, requiring additional direct costs and indirect costs inherent in taking children to the physician's office.

II. Pathogenesis and Epidemiology

Most cold viruses are spread through contact with contaminated surfaces and hand-to-hand contact (15,16). Touching fingers to the nose or eyes gives portals of entry to the host. Certain viruses are also spread as infectious aerosols, generated by sneezing or coughing (17,18). Additionally, certain viruses appear to be more common in children than adults, such as the respiratory syncytial virus (RSV). However, in general, the same viruses are found in both adults and children, and include rhinoviruses (representing more than 30% of colds), coronaviruses, parainfluenza viruses, adenoviruses, or even influenza strains (19,20). Seasonal variations in the incidence of colds is apparent. Generally, there are fewer colds in the warm summer months and more colds during periods of crowding, especially when children start back to school.

The typical incubation period for a cold virus is 24 to 72 hours, but viral shedding can last up to 3 weeks (21). Subjects experimentally infected with rhinovirus may be able to detect the onset of symptoms as early as 16 hours after viral challenge (22). Viral neutralizing antibody, usually of the IgA class, appears in nasal secretions 2 to 3 weeks after infection, at about the same time neutralizing antibody is detected in the serum (23–25). Changes in the peripheral white blood cell count may have pathogenetic significance. Infected, subjects who are not ill have no change in WBC counts, while increase in these counts are seen in infected symptomatic individuals (26). Clinical manifestations of the cold include runny nose, sneezing, cough, nasal stuffiness, and sore throat. Children may experience fevers to a moderate degree, and the nasal discharge may change from clear to purulent.

Systemic symptoms are less common with most cold viruses than with the influenza virus. Influenza virus is associated with muscle aches, malaise, and headaches. If fever, purulent drainage, postnasal drip, and cough last beyond 5 days, a secondary bacterial infection should be suspected. Malaise or facial pain might suggest secondary sinusitis. Dyspnea or overt asthma may be indicative of lung involvement. In fact, bronchial hyperreactivity, secondary to a cold, can last for weeks (27–29). Asthma and chronic obstructive pulmonary disease (COPD) typically exacerbate during a URI (30,31), so what can be a trivial illness to some might represent a life-threatening problem to others.

In children, otitis media is a frequent bacterial complication of the common cold, generally presenting late in the course of an illness and accompanied by diminished hearing and/or ear pain.

Contributing or exacerbating factors of a cold include psychological stress (32) and smoking (33). In fact, smokers appear to be at greater risk first for developing infections, and second for suffering more severe symptoms than nonsmokers. Additionally, in children, exposure to second-hand smoke is not only associated with an increased risk of URI, but with persistent wheezing (34–36) as well as with bronchial hyperreactivity (37,38).

Patients on corticosteroids, especially those taking high doses of these agents, also may be at an increased risk for developing cold infections (39). Aspirin and acetaminophen may suppress seroneutralizing antibodies, and are thereby associated with continued nasal signs and symptoms. A trend toward a longer period of viral shedding has been noted in association with both these agents (40).

Inflammatory medications are thought to contribute to many of the symptoms seen with upper respiratory infections. Although most studies find no histamine in nasal secretions (26,41), some investigators find them in a subgroup of normal subjects, especially in subjects with a history of allergic rhinitis following rhinovirus inoculations (42).

Kinins, such as bradykinin, and interleukins such as IL-1β, IL-6, and IL-8, have been found in nasal secretions of experimentally in rhinovirus infection (26,43,44), yet their exact role in the pathogenesis is still unclear.

Neurologic factors play a role by control of glandular secretions. The rhinorrhea seen especially during the latter stages of the illness is under control of cholinergic neurologic pathways (42). Neurologic pathways are also associated with the hyperreactivity of the airways associated with rhinovirus infections (45,46).

III. Management of the Common Cold

A. Nonpharmacologic or OTC Remedies

Almost every culture has a favorite "home remedy" for the treatment of the common cold. Chicken soup is still the favorite home remedy, and has actually been demonstrated to improve mucociliary clearance (47). A hot lemon tea "toddy" might be a close second in popularity, served with or without honey. Various spices, onions, goose grease, castor oil, potatoes, vinegar, and even sulfur and molasses have their advocates; however, there is very little literature to support their effectiveness. Vitamin C may decrease the duration of cold symptoms (48,49), but it continues to be a controversial choice of therapy. Although data from one review article (49) suggest a 20% reduction in symptom intensity and duration in some patients who were given 2 g or more vitamin C per day, other studies relate no beneficial effect or only a slight antihistamine/anticholinergic effect of the vitamin (50,51).

While there are published studies (52,53) advocating the effectiveness of heated, humidified air for the relief of infectious rhinitis symptoms, no benefits have been demonstrated in patients with the common cold in other randomized controlled trials (54–56). With this modality, one must also be concerned about the possible risk of injury to children, since scalding and burns can occur. Some authors do report a connection between regular sauna bathing and a decreased incidence of the common cold (57).

B. Pharmacologic Remedies

Zinc Lozenges

Recently, there has been a lot of enthusiasm over the use of zinc gluconate lozenges. When taken every 2 hours while awake, these compounds have been reported to reduce the duration of common cold symptoms. Despite the beneficial effect described, there are greater side effects in the group treated with zinc than in the placebo group, manifested by nausea and "bad taste" (58). A review of the literature (59–61) points to at least three studies which demonstrated the beneficial effect of these lozenges, and four that did not. In fact, in a meta-analysis of trials with zinc lozenges for the common cold, the authors concluded that evidence was still lacking for their use (62).

Analgesic/Anti-Inflammatory Agents

Fever, headaches, and muscle pains are often treated with aspirin or acetaminophen. Surprisingly, such compounds may have a detrimental effect on the common cold by actually decreasing blood levels of "good" neutralizing antibodies and possibly increasing viral shedding (40). Naproxen has not been demonstrated to reduce the production of neutralizing antibodies, but it has not been shown to increase them, either. Sperber and colleagues (63) showed that naproxen did appear to help in the relief of such symptoms as headache, malaise, myalgia, and cough, but these investigators could not demonstrate any evidence to show that the agent alters the cold's course of viral shedding. Aspirin is not the treatment of choice in infants and children because of the risk of Reye's syndrome associated with its use.

Antitussives

In general, cough suppressants have minimal effectiveness in children who are younger than 2 years of age (64). Moreover, in children and many adults, cough may more successfully be treated with bronchodilator types of medication. If bronchodilators have been tried and sleep is disturbed, or daily activities are compromised, dextromethorphan, 10 to 20 mg every 4 hours, or 30 mg every 6 to 8 hours, can be used in adults.

Antihistamines

The role of antihistamines in relief of symptoms associated with the common cold has long been debated. The symptoms of sneezing and rhinorrhea may well abate with administration of the sedating, first-generation antihistamines, but this response is thought to be due to the anticholinergic properties of the drugs in this class—not the antagonism of histamine (65). Furthermore, although the first-generation antihistamines are known to produce sedation, the detrimental effect of this on cold sufferers' performance and behavior is often not fully appreciated. For adults and children, the abundant oversupply of the over-the-counter antihistamine preparations available poses a potential for serious impairment—at work and at school. Typically, drugs in this class do not relieve the symptoms of sore throat and nasal obstruction (66–68). Although most of the non- or low-sedating antihistamines, such as astemizole, cetirizine, and loratadine, have not been studied for the common cold, terfenadine has been reported to be relatively ineffective in relief of symptoms (69,70).

Decongestants

Review of data from clinical trials published between 1950 and 1991 confirms the ineffectiveness of antihistamines for treating colds (8). Decongestant agents generally relieve congestion; however, their effectiveness varies (71,72). Oral forms are preferred over topical agents, which have been associated with significant rebound congestion or worsening of symptoms (73). Topical nasal decongestants may provide some relief from congestive nasal symptoms in patients with the common cold (67,74), but their effect usually does not carry over to the other symptoms of a cold, such as cough, earache, or rhinorrhea, or do anything about preventing complications such as sinus disease or otitis media (75,76). Their use in infants is contraindicated, mainly because of their rebound effects.

Additionally, the general side effects associated with over-the-counter decongestants are a major consideration when weighing their potential for effectiveness in treatment of the common cold. Side effects of decongestants can be mild, and include jitteriness or irritability. Occasionally, they can be bizarre and serious, such as visual hallucinations or psychosis (77–79).

Antihistamine/Decongestant Combinations

Hutton and coworkers (80) examined the effectiveness of an antihistamine/decongestant combination, used in preschool children with common colds.

They found no clinically significant improvement of symptoms after 48 hours of therapy. Combination products that contain analgesics may very well improve symptoms such as cough, sore throat, and aches (81). Apparently an antihistamine-decongestant/antitussive combination is superior to an antihistamine/expectorant combination, according to various European investigators (82). Godomski and Horton found a reduction in nasal symptoms and signs at day three and five of the illness, with minimal side effects. Overdoses of combination products may produce serious complications, as described after an infant less than 2 years of age ingested a combination of dextromethorphan, an antihistamine, and a decongestant (82). Thus, combination products in infants should be used with great caution.

Ipratropium Bromide

In many countries outside the United States, ipratropium bromide exists as a pressurized aerosol. Studies have confirmed its usefulness in the treatment of the common cold (83,84). Typically, watery rhinorrhea is ameliorated, with the beneficial effect occurring during the first days of the cold (83).

Østberg et al. (84) gave a high dose of ipratropium bromide pressurized aerosol (400 µg four times a day) to define the maximal benefit expected from an anticholinergic therapy. Symptom scores and secretion weights were reduced 56% and 58%, respectively. It reduced the watery secretions but not the mucopurulent secretions. The high dose was associated with dryness in the nose and mouth in many patients (84).

Using an experimental model of rhinorrhea induced by nasal methacholine challenge, Becher and coworkers suggested that ipratroprium bromide could be given less than four times daily since there was a significant effect demonstrable for 12 hours with 40 µg and for 18 hours with 80 µg ipratropium bromide micronized powder (85).

In many countries, the aqueous form of ipratropium bromide has been employed successfully in the treatment of rhinorrhea secondary to allergic or nonallergic rhinitis. For the common cold, the dose is two sprays in each nostril of the 0.06% concentration, given three to four times per day. Ipratropium bromide nasal spray, in doses of 42 to 168 µg per nostril, given three to four times daily in patients with naturally acquired colds, reduced rhinorrhea and even had a slight effect on congestion, along with subjective assessment scores (86,87). Adverse effects were primarily dose-related, and the events most frequently reported were nasal dryness and blood-tinged mucus (in up to 70% of patients).

In a multicenter double-blind placebo-controlled trial of 411 patients aged 14 to 50 years, there was a significant reduction of rhinorrhea and sneezing associated with the dose of two 42-µg sprays per nostril, given three to four times per day. Again, the side effect reported as occurring most frequently in the treatment group was blood-tinged mucus. This was evident in 16.8% of patients, as compared to 3.6% of patients in the control group receiving a saline placebo (88).

Anti-Inflammatory Agents

Cromolyn and nedocromil have been employed with mixed results (89,90). Their safety record is excellent. One study of intranasally administered nedocromil showed improvement in performance impairment (91). When both intranasal and inhaled sodium cromolyn were given after symptoms of a cold began, improvement was noted—mainly in lower respiratory symptoms (92). These agents are characterized by good safety profiles, also.

Intranasal or systemic steroids may suppress inflammation during the first days of infection, and their use would seem to merit further investigation (93).

Antibiotics

It is not uncommon for physicians to prescribe an antibiotic for the treatment of colds, even though a secondary infection such as otitis media or sinusitis is not diagnosed. Investigators assessing the prescribing behavior of family practitioners reported that 60% of these physicians prescribed an antibiotic, despite coding on their outpatient encounter form solely that the patient had a URI of a viral nature (12).

This practice is inappropriate, except perhaps in small children and maybe in allergic patients who already may have compromised local anatomy due to swelling, which can contribute to the development of secondary bacterial infection. The antibiotic chosen should, ideally, cover the most commonly encountered organisms, such as *Moraxella catarrhalis* or *Haemophilus influenzae*, with a relatively high incidence of beta-lactamase-producing organisms, and *Streptococcus pneumoniae* with emerging resistance due to other mechanisms.

Even in cold patients with evidence of ostial obstruction by computerized tomography (CT) (94), only 2% to 5% actually develop secondary bacterial sinusitis (95,96).

C. Investigational Therapy

Interferon

Interferon has been administered by the nasal route in most clinical trials set up to determine its effectiveness in the treatment of URIs. The agent has proven most efficacious when given shortly before or after exposure to the virus, and also when given prophylactically to potential contacts in family outbreaks (97–100). Unfortunately, there are a number of drawbacks to the use of interferon: it is expensive to produce, requires frequent dosing, and does not reliably produce consistent results. The type of interferon used can make a difference when assessing efficacy, too. Beta and gamma interferon have proven disappointing in treatment of symptoms associated with URIs, for example, as opposed to interferon alpha-2b (101).

A combination therapy of intranasal interferon alpha 2b, ipratropium bromide 80 µg, inhaled three times per day, and oral naproxen, 250 mg three times per day, was shown to reduce cold symptoms significantly in the 27 adults studied after experimental rhinovirus infection in a placebo-controlled study (102,103). The therapy was started 24 hours after experimental inoculation and continued for 4 days. The symptomatic improvement was accompanied by reduced viral shedding.

Antiviral Agents

Currently available antiviral agents, e.g., amantadine, have been less help than hoped for in the treatment of symptoms associated with the common cold. The intercellular adhesion molecule ICAM-1 is a receptor for 90% of the rhinoviruses (104). It is not surprising that the ICAM receptor antagonist agents are under active investigation, since they may block the virus from binding to the host cell (103,105,106). The development of synthetic agents, or monoclonal antibodies, to block the receptor has the potential to prevent the most frequently culpable cold viruses from infecting cells (66,107). However, to date, these agents have yet to be studied in large-scale clinical trials. More experience is needed before definitive assessments can be made. Pirodavin, a virus capable binding agent, does not ameliorate established infection, but it may serve as a preventive agent (108,109).

IV. Prevention

Vaccine programs for respiratory viruses have met with limited success. The influenza vaccine has proven effective, but it is costly and must be given annually, due to the antigenic shifts. More to the point: it does not provide protection against infectious agents associated with the common cold.

Vaccines against RSV have been associated with unwanted and unexpected side effects, and are not now being utilized. Rhinoviruses are very difficult targets for vaccine designs, since there are well over 100 different stereotypes.

Since most colds are transmitted through hand contact from the virus on surfaces, and then self-inoculated to the nose or eyes, the spread could be slowed by frequent hand washing, as well as better education. Sometimes, though, the infectious culprit is via aerosol, borne by an infectious person's sneeze or cough. So, although completely avoiding people who are coughing and sneezing is probably the best preventive medicine, it is hardly practical.

Attempts have been made to impregnate virucidal materials into facial tissues, but such efforts have been shown not to be of much value over the long term in large populations (110–113).

V. Conclusion

When it comes to treatment of the common cold, certainly, more progress has been made since William Osler's assertion: "There is just one way to treat a cold, i.e., with contempt." Still, the common cold continues to charge a high price to society: in direct costs such as drug acquisition costs and days lost from work and school, and in indirect costs, such as those associated with behavioral impairment—and oftentimes overlooked—but very real side effects of many of the over-the-counter cold preparations available.

Also, patients pay very high prices for antibiotic prescriptions which have dubious value in helping halt the course of their viral URIs. The practice of overprescribing antibiotics may ultimately have the opposite effect and wind up lowering patients' resistance to opportunistic bacteria.

In patients with asthma or COPD, or other existing respiratory maladies, the common cold poses a potentially serious problem, giving rise to the possibility of acute exacerbations of patients' underlying disease.

Results have been mixed in practice with agents used in treatment of common colds. In controlled clinical trials, the anticholinergic agent ipratropium bromide has proven effective in relief of rhinorrhea associated with the common cold. Some clinical experience with anti-inflammatory agents, such as cromolyn and nedocromil, has been promising. Over-the-counter cold medications have become household staples in self-medicating, but the actual data on their effectiveness are limited and weak, especially in children. Zinc and vitamin C are frequently employed in self-treatment of the common cold, with varying reports of success.

There is a need for carefully designed, randomized studies of agents focused on clinically useful, specific benefits—such as lessening of nasal discharge and relief of coughing—in treatment of the common cold. Careful consideration should be given to appropriate dosing and potentially serious side effects in different age groups. Finally, there must be a large scale effort to educate patients about how to protect themselves against the spread of the common cold infection. Frequent hand washing and reasonable avoidance of persons already infected are a must. These simple precautions go a long way toward keeping more of us healthy.

References

1. Sperber SJ, Levine PA, Sorrentino JV, Riker DK, Hayden FG. Ineffectiveness of recombinant interferon-beta serine nasal drops for prophylaxis of natural colds. J Infect Dis 1989; 160:700–705.
2. Dingle JH, Badger GF, Jordan WS Jr. Illness in the Home: A Study of 25,000 Illnesses in a Group of Cleveland Families. Cleveland, OH: Cleveland Care Writers Reserve, University Press 1964:33–96.
3. Gwaltney JM Jr, Henley JO, Simon G, Jordan WS Jr. Rhinovirus infections in an industrial population. I. The occurrence of illness. N Engl J Med 1966; 275: 1261–1268.
4. US Department of Health and Human Services. Health Care Finan Rev. 1992; 14:1–30.
5. Gwaltney J. The common cold. In: Mandell G, Douglas R, Bennett, J, eds. Principles and Practices of Infectious Disease. New York. Churchill Livingstone, 1990:439–493.
6. Koster F. Respiratory infections. In: Barker LR, Burton JR, Zieve PD, eds. Principles of Ambulatory Medicine. Baltimore: Williams & Wilkins, 1987: 347–355.
7. Benson V, Marano MA. Current estimates from the National Health Interview Survey, 1993. Vital Health Stat 10 (189). Hyattsville, MD: National Center for Health Statistics, 1994.
8. Smith MBH, Feldman W. Over-the-counter cold medications: a critical review of clinical trials between 1950 and 1991. JAMA 1993; 269:2258–2263.
9. Kogan MD, Pappas G, Yu SM, Kotelchuck M. Over-the-counter medication use among US preschool-age children. JAMA 1994; 272:1025–1030.
10. English JA, Bauman KA. Evidence-based management of upper respiratory infection in a family practice teaching clinic. Fam Med 1997; 29:38–41.
11. Meltzer EO, Tyrell RJ, Rich D, Wood C. A pharmacologic continuum in the

treatment of rhinorrhea: the clinician as economist. J Allergy Clin Immunol 1994; 95:1147–1152.
12. Mainous AG, Hueston WJ, Clark JR. Antibiotics and upper respiratory infection: do some folks think there is a cure for the common cold? J Fam Pract 1996; 42:357–361.
13. Red Book; Pharmacy's Fundamental Reference. Montvale, JH: Medical Economics Data Production Company, 1994:100.
14. Holt E, Guyer B, Hughart N, et al. The contribution of missed opportunities to childhood underimmunization in Baltimore. Pediatrics 1996; 97:474–480.
15. Sattar SA, Jacobsen H, Springthorpe VS, Cusack TM, Rubino JR. Chemical disinfection interrupt transfer rhinovirus type 14 from environmental surfaces to hands. Appl Environ Microbiol 1993; 59:1579–1585.
16. Ansari SA, Springthorpe VS, Sattar SA, Rivard S, Rahman M. Potential role of hands in the spread of respiratory viral infections: studies with human parainfluenza virus 3 and rhinovirus 14. J Clin Microbiol 1991; 29:2115–2119.
17. Dick EC, Jennings LC, Mink KA, et al. Aerosol transmission of rhinovirus colds. J Infect Dis 1987; 156:442–448.
18. Hendley JO, Gwaltney JM Jr. Mechanisms of transmission of rhinovirus infections. Epidemiol Rev 1988; 10:242–258.
19. Glezen WP. The common cold. In: Gorbach SL, Bartlett JG, Blacklow NR, eds. Infectious Disease. Philadelphia: W.B. Saunders, 1992:455–460.
20. Spector SL. The common cold: current therapy and natural history. J Allergy Clin Immunol 1995; 95:1133–1138.
21. Winther B, Gwaltney JM Jr, Mygind N, et al. Sites of rhinovirus recovery after point inoculation of the upper airway. JAMA 1986; 256:1763–1767.
22. Harris JM II, Gwaltney JM Jr. Incubation periods of experimental rhinovirus infection and illness. J Infect Dis 1996; 23:1287–1290.
23. Hendley JO, Edmonson WP Jr, Gwaltney JM Jr. Relationship between naturally acquired immunity and infection of two rhinoviruses in volunteers. J Infect Dis 1972; 125:243–248.
24. Cate TR, Rossen RD, Douglas R Jr, et al. The role of nasal secretion and serum antibody in the rhinovirus common cold. Am J Epidemiol 1996; 84:352–363.
25. Rossen RD, Kasel JA, Couch RB. The secretory immune system: its relation to respiratory viral infection. Prog Med Virol 1971; 13:194–238.
26. Naclerio RM, Proud D, Lichtenstein LM, et al. Kinins are generated during experimental rhinovirus colds. J Infect Dis 1988; 157:133–142.
27. Johnston SL, Pattermore PK, Sanderson G, et al. Community study of role of viral infections in exacerbations of asthma in 9- to 11-year-old children. GMJ 1995; 310:1225–1228.
28. Bardin PG, Fraenkel D, Sanderson G, et al. Increased sensitivity to the consequences of rhinoviral infection in atopic subjects. Chest 1995; 107(3 suppl):S157.
29. Fraenkel DJ, Bardin PG, Sanderson G, et al. Lower airway inflammation during rhinovirus colds in normal and in asthmatic subjects. Am J Respir Crit Care Med 1995; 151:879–886.

30. Spector SL, Nicklas R, eds. Practice parameters for the diagnosis and treatment of asthma. J Allergy Clin Immunol 1995; 96:707–870.
31. Spector SL. Asthma and chronic obstructive lung disease: a pharmacologic approach. Disease-a-Month 1991; 37(1).
32. Stone AA, Bovbjerg DH, Neale JM, et al. Development of common cold symptoms following experimental rhinovirus infection is related to prior stressful life events. Behav Med 1992; 18:115–120.
33. Cohen S, Tyrrell DA, Russell MA, Jarvis MJ, Smith AP. Smoking, alcohol consumption, and susceptibility to the common cold. Am J Public Health 1993; 83:1277–1283.
34. Cogswell JI, Mitchell EB, Alexander J. Parental smoking, breast feeding, and respiratory infections in development of allergic disease. Arch Dis Child 1987; 62:238.
35. Fergusson DM, Horwood LJ, Shannon FT. Parental smoking and respiratory illness in infancy. Arch Dis Child 1980; 55:358.
36. Burchfiel CM, Higgins MW, Keller JB, et al. Passive smoking in childhood respiratory conditions and pulmonary function in Tecumseh, Michigan. Am Rev Repir Dis 1986; 133:966.
37. Murray AB, Morrison BJ. The effect of cigarette smoke from the mother on bronchial responsiveness and severity of symptoms in children with asthma. J Allergy Clin Immunol 1986; 575:77.
38. Martinez FD, Antognoni G, Macri F, et al. Parental smoking enhances bronchial responsiveness in nine-year-old children. Am Rev Respir Dis 1988; 138:518.
39. Oehling AG, Akdis CA, Schapowal A, Blaser K, Schmitz M, Simon HU. Suppression of the immune system by oral glucocorticoid therapy in bronchial asthma. Allergy 1997; 52:144–154.
40. Graham NM, Burrell CJ, Douglas RM, Debelle P, Davies L. Adverse effects of aspirin, acetaminophen, and ibuprofen on immune function, viral shedding, and clinical status in rhinovirus-infected volunteers. J Infect Dis 1990; 162:1277–1282.
41. Eggleston PA, Hendley JO, Gwaltney JM Jr, et al. Mediation of immediate hyperreactivity in nasal secretions during natural colds and rhinovirus infections. Acta Otolaryngol Suppl 1984; 413:25–35.
42. Igarashi Y, Skomer DP, Doyle WJ, et al. Analysis of nasal secretions during experimental rhinovirus upper respiratory infections. J Allergy Clin Immunol 1993; 92:722–731.
43. Proud D, Gwaltney JM Jr, Hendley JD, et al. Increased levels of interleukins-1 are detected in nasal secretions of volunteers during experimental rhinovirus colds. J Infect Dis 1994; 169:1007–1013.
44. Zhu Z, Tang W, Roy A, et al. Rhinovirus stimulation of interleukin-6 in vivo and in vitro evidence for nuclear factor KB-dependent transcription activation. J Clin Invest 1996; 97:421–430.
45. Aguilina AT, Hall WJ, Douglas RG Jr, Utell MJ. Airway reactivity in subjects with viral upper respiratory tract infections: the effect of exercise and colds. Am Rev Respir Dis 1980; 122:3–10.
46. Empey DW, Laitinen LA, Jacobs L, et al. Mechanisms of bronchial hyperreac-

tivity in normal subjects after upper respiratory infections. Am Rev Respir Dis 1976; 113:131–139.
47. Saketkhoo K, Januszkiewicz A, Sackner M. Effects of drinking hot water, cold water, and chicken soup on nasal mucus velocity and nasal airflow resistance. Chest 1978; 74:408.
48. Hemila H. Vitamin C and the common cold. Br J Nutr 1992; 67:3–16.
49. Hemila H. Does vitamin C alleviate the symptoms of the common cold? A review of current evidence. Scand J Infect Dis 1994; 26:1–6.
50. Dykes MH, Meier P. Ascorbic acid and the common cold: evaluation of its efficiency and toxicity. JAMA 1975; 231:1073–1079.
51. Burns JJ, Rivers JM, Machlin LJ, et al., eds. Proceedings of a recent symposium on advances in understanding of vitamin C metabolism. Ann NY Acad Sci 1987; 498.
52. Ophir D, Elad Y. Effects of steam inhalation on nasal patency and nasal symptoms in patients with the common cold. Am J Otoloaryngol 1987; 8:149–153.
53. Tyrrell D, Barrow I, Arthur J. Local hyperthermia benefits natural and experimental common colds [published erratum appears in BMJ 1989; 299:600]. GMJ 1989; 298:1280–1283.
54. Macknin ML, Mathew S, Medendorp SV. Effect of inhaling heated vapor on symptoms of the common cold. JAMA 1990; 264:989–991.
55. Forstall GJ, Macknin ML, Yen-Lieberman BR, et al. Effect of inhaling heated vapor on symptoms of the common cold. JAMA 1994; 271:1109–1111.
56. Hendley JO, Abbot RD, Beasley PP, et al. Effect of inhalation of hot humidified air on experimental rhinovirus infection [see comments]. JAMA 1994; 271: 1112–1113. [Comment in JAMA 1994; 271:1122–1124.]
57. Ernst E, Pecho E, Wirz P, Saradeth T. Regular sauna bathing and the incidence of common colds. Ann Med 1990; 22:225–227.
58. Mossad SB, Macknin M, Medendorp SV, et al. Zinc gluconate lozenges for treating the common cold: a randomized, double-blind, placebo-controlled study. Ann Intern Med 1996;125:81–88. [Editorial comment in Ann Intern Med 1996; 125:142–144.]
59. Godfrey JC. Zinc for the common cold [letter]. Antimicrob Agents Chemother 1988; 32:605–606.
60. Eby GA. Stability constants of zinc complexes affect common cold treatment results [letter]. Antimicrob Agents Chemother 1988; 32:606–607.
61. Zarembo JE, Godfrey JC, Godfrey JM Jr. Zinc (II) in saliva: determination of concentrations produced by different formulations of zinc gluconate lozenges containing common excipients. J Pharm Sci 1992; 81:128–130.
62. Jackson JL, Peterson C, Lesko E. A meta-analysis of zinc salts lozenges and the common cold. Arch Intern Med 1997; 157:2373–2376.
63. Sperber SJ, Hendley JO, Hayden FG, et al. Effects of naproxen on experimental rhinovirus colds: a randomized, double-blind, controlled trial. Ann Intern Med 1992; 117:37–41.

64. Taylor JA, Novack AH, Almquist JR, et al. Efficacy of cough suppressants in children. J Pediatr 1993; 122:799–802.
65. Sperber SJ, Hayden FG. Chemotherapy of rhinovirus colds. Antimicrob Agents Chemother 1988; 32:409–419.
66. Gaffey MJ, Kaiser DL, Hayden FG. Ineffectiveness of oral terfenadine in natural colds: evidence against histamine as a mediator of common cold symptoms. Pediatr Infect Dis J 1988; 7(3):223–228.
67. Lowenstein SR, Parrino TA. Management of common cold. Adv Intern Med 1987; 32:207–233.
68. Gaffey MJ, Gwaltney JM Jr, Sastre A, et al. Intranasally and orally administered antihistamine treatment of experimental rhinovirus colds. Am Rev Respir Dis 1987:135:556–560.
69. Berkowitz RB, Tinkleman DG. Evaluation of oral terfenadine for treatment of the common cold. Ann Allergy 1991; 67:593–597.
70. Gaffey MJ, Karen DL, Hayden FG. Ineffectiveness of oral terfenadine in natural colds: evidence against histamines as a mediator of common cold symptoms. J Infect Dis 1988; 7:233–238.
71. Fireman P. Pathophysiology and pharmacotherapy of common upper respiratory diseases. Pharmacotherapy 1993; 13:101S–109S, 143S–146S.
72. West S, Brandon B, Stolley P, et al. Review of antihistamines and the common cold. Pediatrics 1975; 56:100–107.
73. Hendeles L. Selecting a decongestant. Pharmacotherapy 1993; 13(6 pt 2): 129S–134S.
74. Lea P. Double-blind controlled evaluation of nasal decongestant effect of day nurse in the common cold. J Intern Med Res 1984; 12:124–127.
75. Akerlund A, Klint T, Olen L, et al. Nasal decongestant effect of oxymetazoline in the common cold: an objective dose-response study in 106 patients. J Laryngol Otol 1989; 103:743–746.
76. Cantekin EL, Mandel EM, Bluestone CD, et al. Lack of efficacy of decongestant-antihistamine combination for otitis media with effusion (secretory otitis media) in children. Results of a double-blind, randomized trial. N Engl J Med 1983; 308:297–301.
77. Sills JA, Nunn AJ, Sankey RJ. Visual hallucinations in children receiving decongestants [letter]. BMJ [Clin Res] 1984; 288(6434):1912–1913.
78. Orson J, Bassow L. Over-the-counter cough formulas. Clin Pediatr 1987; 26: 287–288.
79. Kane FJ, Green BQ. Psychotic episodes associated with the use of common proprietary decongestants. Am J Psychiatry 1966; 123:484–487.
80. Hutton N, Wilson MH, Mellits ED, et al. Effectiveness of an antihistamine-decongestant combination for young children with the common cold: randomized, controlled clinical trial. J Pediatr 1991; 118:125–130.
81. Weipple G. Therapeutic approaches to the common cold in children. Clin Ther 1984; 6:475–482.

82. Gadomski A, Horton L. The need for rational therapeutics in the use of cough and cold medicine in infants. Pediatrics 1992; 89(4 pt 2):774–776.
83. Borum P, Olsen L, Winter B, Mygind N. Ipratropium nasal spray: a new treatment for rhinorrhea in the common cold. Am Rev Respir Dis 1981; 123:418–420.
84. Østberg B, Winther B, Borum P. Mygind N. Common cold and high-dose ipratropium bromide: use of anticholinergic medication as an indicator of reflex-mediated hypersecretion. Rhinology 1997.
85. Becker B, Borum S, Nielsen K, Mygind N, Borum P. A time-dose study of the effect of topical ipratropium bromide on methacholine-induced rhinorrhea in patients with perennial non-allergic rhinitis. Clin Otolaryngol 1997; 22:132–134.
86. Dockhorn R, Grossman J, Posner M, et al. A double-blind, placebo-controlled study of the safety and efficacy of ipratropium bromide nasal spray versus placebo in patients with the common cold. J Allergy Clin Immunol 1992; 90:1076–1082.
87. Diamond L, Dockhorn RJ, Grossman J, et al. A dose-response study of the efficacy and safety of ipratropium bromide nasal spray in the treatment of the common cold. J Allergy Clin Immunol 1995; 95:1139–1146.
88. Hayden FG, Diamond L, Wood PB, Korts DC, Wecker MT. Effectiveness and safety of intranasal ipratropium bromide in common colds. Ann Intern Med 1996; 125:89–97.
89. Barrow GI, Higgins PG, al-Nakib W, et al. The effect of intranasal nedocromil sodium on viral upper respiratory tract infections in human volunteers. Clin Exp Allergy 1990; 20:45–51.
90. Sederberg-Olsen JF, Sederberg-Olson AE. Intranasal sodium cromoglycate in post-catarrhal hyperreactive rhino-sinusitis: a double-blind placebo controlled trial. Rhinology 1989; 27:251–255.
91. Konig P, Eigen H, Ellis MH, et al. The effect of nedocromil sodium on childhood asthma during the viral season. Am J Respir Crti Care Med 1995; 152:1879–1886.
92. Farr BM, Gwaltney JM Jr, Hendley JO, et al. A randomized controlled trial of glucocorticoid prophylaxis against experimental rhinovirus infection. J Infect Dis 1990; 162:1173–1177.
93. Johnston SL, Holgate ST. Epidemiology of viral respiratory tract infections. In: Myint S, Taylor-Robinson D, eds. Viral and Other Infections of the Human Respiratory Tract. London: Chapman & Hall, 1996:1–38.
94. Gwaltney JM Jr, Phillips CD, Miller RD, et al. Computed tomographic study of the common cold. N Engl J Med 1994; 330:25–30.
95. Berg O, Carenfelt C, Rystedt G, et al. Occurrence of asymptomatic sinusitis in common cold and other acute ENT infections. Rhinology 1986; 24:223–225.
96. Dingle JH, Badger GF, Jordan WS Jr. Illness in the Home: A Study of 25,000 Illnesses in a Group of Cleveland Families. Cleveland: The Press of Western Reserve University, 1964:347.
97. Hayden FG, Gwaltney JM Jr. Intranasal interferon alpha 2 for prevention of rhinovirus infection and illness. J Infect Dis 1983; 148:543–550.

98. Samo TC, Greenberg SB, Couch RB, et al. Efficacy and tolerance of intranasally applied recombinant leukocyte A interferon in normal volunteers. J Infect Dis 1983; 148:535–542.
99. Hayden FG, Albrecht JK, Kaiser DL, et al. Prevention of natural colds by contact prophylaxis with intranasal alpha 2-interferon. N Engl J Med 1986; 314:71–75.
100. Douglas RM, Moore BW, Miles HB, et al. Prophylactic efficacy of intranasal alpha 2-interferon against rhinovirus infections in the family setting. N Engl J Med 1986; 314:65–70.
101. Higgins PG, al-Nakib W, Barrow GI, et al. Recombinant human interferon-gamma as prophylaxis against rhinovirus colds in volunteers. J Interferon Res 1988; 8:591–596.
102. Sperber SJ, Levine PA, Sorrentino JV, et al. Ineffectiveness of recombinant interferon-beta serine nasal drops for prophylaxis of natural colds. J Infect Dis 1989; 160:700–705.
103. Gwaltney JM Jr. Combined antiviral and antimediator treatment of rhinovirus colds. J Infect Dis 1992; 166:776–782.
104. Cecchin A. The emergency of new clinical clues may bring us closer to a cure for the common cold. Med World News 1993; 30–42.
105. Marlin SD, Stauton DE, Springer TA, et al. A soluble form of intercellular allergic molecule-1 inhibits rhinovirus infection. Nature 1990;344:70–72.
106. Crump CE Jr, Arruda E, Hayden FG. In vitro inhibition activity of soluble ICAM-1 for the numbered serotypes of human rhinovirus. Antiviral Chem 1993; 4:323–327.
107. Johnston SL, Bardin PG, Pattermore PK. Viruses as precipitants of asthma symptoms. III. Rhinoviruses: molecular biology and prospects for future intervention. Clin Exp Allergy 1993; 23:237–246.
108. Barrow GI, Higgens PC, Tyrrell DAJ, Andries K. An appearance of the efficacy of the antiviral R61837 in rhinovirus infections in human volunteers. Antiviral Chem Chemother 1990; 1:279–283.
109. Hayden FG, Andries K, Janssen PA. Safety and efficacy of intranasal Priodavis (R7997S) in experimental rhinovirus infections. Antimicrob Agents Chemother 1992; 36:727–732.
110. Hayden FB, Gwaltney JM Jr, Colonno RJ. Modification of experimental rhinovirus colds by receptor blockade. Antiviral Res 1988; 9:233–247.
111. Dick EC, Hossain SU, Mink KA, et al. Interruption of transmission of rhinovirus colds among human volunteers using virucidal paper handkerchiefs. J Infect Dis 1986; 153:352–356.
112. Longini IM Jr, Monto AS. Efficacy of virucidal nasal tissues in interrupting familial transmission of respiratory agents. A field trial in Tecumseh, Michigan. Am J Epidemiol 1988; 128:639–644.
113. Farr BM, Hendley JO, Kaiser DL, et al. Two randomized controlled trials of virucidal nasal tissues in the prevention of natural upper respiratory infections. Am J Epidemiol 1988; 128:1162–1172.

7

Anticholinergics in Combination Bronchodilator Therapy in COPD

STEPHEN I. RENNARD

University of Nebraska Medical Center
Omaha, Nebraska

I. Introduction

Bronchodilators form one of the mainstays of therapy in patients with chronic obstructive pulmonary disease (COPD). Aggressive use of these agents can often improve lung function in patients with significant symptoms due to respiratory impairment. As a result, patients can often experience both a reduction in symptoms and an improvement in their quality of life even if bronchodilators are only partially effective in improving expiratory airflow. Since bronchodilators are available in several classes, it is obviously of clinical interest to determine if combination therapy with several bronchodilators might have clinical advantages. This chapter will review combination bronchodilator therapy focusing on patients with COPD and on the role of anticholinergics in such combinations.

II. Bronchodilators and Expiratory Airflow Limitation

In asthma, episodic contraction of airway smooth muscle results in intermittent narrowing of the airways (1). This can often result in the acute limitation of airflow that characterizes asthma attacks. Other mechanisms such as airway edema (2) and accumulation of airway secretions (3) can also contribute to airflow limitation in asthma. Nevertheless, airway smooth muscle contraction is felt to be the major contributor to airflow limitation, particularly in patients with mild to moderate disease. As a result, agents that relax airway smooth muscle can have a beneficial effect in asthma, often reversing airflow limitation to normal.

In patients with chronic obstructive pulmonary disease, a variety of mechanisms contribute to expiratory airflow limitation (4). In emphysema, loss of lung elastic recoil both decreases driving pressure and can result in collapse of small airways during forced exhalation. In chronic obstructive bronchitis, inflammation and fibrosis can result in narrowing of small airways due to the accumulation of scarlike material. Airway narrowing due to bronchial smooth muscle contraction can also play a role in COPD, however. As a result, bronchodilators can result in improved airflow in patients with COPD. Because mechanisms other than smooth muscle contraction contribute to airflow limitation, however, the reversibility of airflow limitation in patients with COPD is only partial.

The beta agonist bronchodilators directly result in airway smooth muscle relaxation. They do so by interacting with beta-2 adrenergic receptors on the airway smooth muscle cell surface (5). These receptors, in turn, through G, proteins result in increases in airway smooth muscle cyclic AMP which, in turn, causes a redistribution of intracellular calcium and can induce a contracted smooth muscle to relax. A variety of beta agonists have proved to be clinically useful. Because beta receptors with different specificities are present on other cells, agents most commonly used in current-day practice are those that are relatively specific for the beta-2 receptors present in airway smooth muscle. It is possible that some of the clinical benefits of beta agonists, including beta-2 selective drugs, are partially due to response at these other sites, for example, airway nerves (1,5).

The magnitude of reversibility to beta agonists in patients with COPD is, generally, much less than the reversibility observed in patients with similar airflow limitation who have asthma. While a number of approaches have been made to define "responders," in general a 15% improvement above baseline lung function is regarded as a positive response. Interestingly, the percentage of patients with COPD who respond to a beta agonist bronchodilator increases with the severity of the disease (6). This is, in part, due to the fact that the magnitude of the bronchodilator response is similar in patients with mild airflow limitation and in those with severe airflow limitation. On the other hand, a 200-mL improvement in FEV_1 can represent an insignificant 6.6% improvement in a patient with a 3-L FEV_1 while the same 200-mL improvement can represent a significant 20% improvement in a patient starting with a 1-L FEV_1. This increasing benefit observed from bronchodilators as COPD worsens has been observed both across several studies and within individual studies (6–11).

Theophylline preparations have been widely used in the treatment of patients with chronic obstructive pulmonary disease. Theophylline prevents the breakdown of cyclic AMP by inhibiting the enzyme phosphodiesterase, which converts cyclic AMP to AMP (12). As a result, theophylline is believed to cause improved airflow by inducing smooth muscle relaxation through increases in cyclic AMP similar to beta agonists. Since theophylline and beta agonists affect cyclic AMP by differing mechanisms, their use in combination has been generally regarded as rational. Consistent with this, improved clinical benefit from the combination of beta agonists and theophylline has been reported in a number of trials (13–21). Whether these benefits could be achieved with maximal doses of beta agonists also remains controversial, however. Some of the benefits of theophylline, interestingly, may be due to effects on tissues other than airway smooth muscle. In this regard, theophylline has been noted to have a number of potentially beneficial effects in COPD including diaphragmatic contractility (22), improved mucociliary clearance (23), and effects on the cardiovascular system (24).

Anticholinergic bronchodilators function by blocking endogenous cholinergic tone. Specifically, vagal innervation of the airway can result in airway smooth muscle contraction. Acetylcholine can play several roles along this pathway, being responsible both as the ganglionic neurotransmitter, a function mediated through the M_1 muscarinic receptor, and as the neurotransmitter at the neuromuscular junction that, through the M_3 muscarinic receptor, leads to smooth muscle contraction. Another muscarinic receptor, the M_2 receptor, is present on the postganglionic neuron where it can function as a feedback inhibitor of acetylcholine release. Anticholinergic bronchodilators are believed to prevent smooth muscle contraction primarily by blocking the M_3 receptor at the neuromuscular junction, although an effect at the M_1 receptor may also be beneficial. Interestingly, inhibition of the M_2 receptor might be regarded as detrimental, leading to the possibility that selective muscarinic antagonists may have clinical benefits.

A number of studies have demonstrated that cholinergic tone contributes to airflow limitation in patients with COPD (10,25–28). As a result, anticholinergic drugs are associated with improved airflow in these patients. As with beta agonist bronchodilators, the percentage of patients who respond to anticholinergics appears to increase with increasing severity of disease (7,10,11,29). Also similar to beta agonists, there may also be significant day-to-day variability in responsiveness, perhaps due to variations in cholinergic tone (6,27). This variability in responsiveness (30,31) can confound estimates of best response. While some studies suggest that either beta agonists or anticholinergics may be more effective as bronchodilators in patients with COPD, most studies find that these agents have a similar magnitude of effect. A number of lines of evidence, however, suggest it is rational to combine bronchodilators.

III. Rationale for Combined Bronchodilator Therapy

A. General Considerations

The various classes of bronchodilators (beta agonists, phosphodiesterase inhibitors, and anticholinergics) result in bronchodilatation through differing mechanisms (Fig. 1). It is therefore rational that their combination may be more effective than individual drugs alone. In addition, bronchodilators may affect smooth muscle in different parts of the airways differentially. Specifically, the proximal large airways appear to be more richly endowed with cholinergic receptors (32) and presumably are more affected by anticholinergic bronchodilators (33) than the more peripheral small airways, which are more richly endowed with beta receptors (32) and appear to be more responsive to beta agonists (33). The various drugs used as bronchodilators, moreover, have different pharmacokinetics. This therefore raises the possibility that combined therapy may have advantages with respect to onset or duration of action.

As noted above, various bronchodilators may have effects outside the airways. Such effects could also be beneficial in combination. Finally, while many physiological studies, both in vivo and in vitro, are designed to evaluate the acute effects of bronchodilators on smooth muscle tone, long-term effects may be slightly different. In this regard, tachyphylaxis, that is, loss of effectiveness with continued use, may be a particular problem in COPD patients. Specifically, patients with COPD, by definition (34), have some degree of irreversible airflow limitation and will therefore generally require continuing

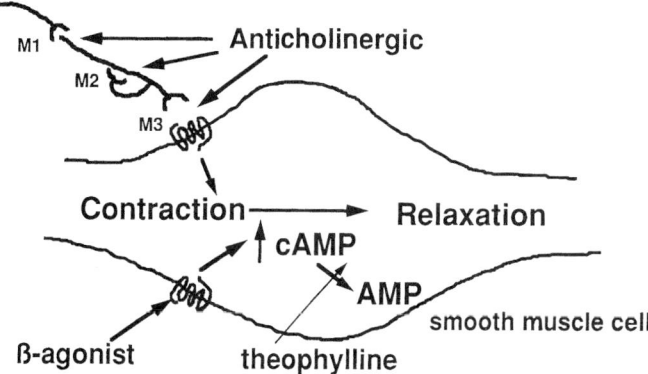

Figure 1 Different classes of bronchodilators interact with smooth muscle cells through different mechanisms. Beta agonists interact with a membrane receptor, leading to increases in intracellular cyclic AMP. Theophylline can increase cyclic AMP by blocking its breakdown by phosphodiesterase to AMP. Anticholinergics block the effect of acetylcholine. The M_3 receptor on the surface of airway smooth muscle, when activated, leads to airway contraction. In addition to differences in mechanism of action, various bronchodilators can differ with respect to pharmacokinetics, site of action within the airway, long-term effects, and effects on tissues other than airway. (See text for details.)

regular therapy with bronchodilators. Combination may have advantages for the long-term treatment required clinically.

Many studies have been conducted to evaluate whether a combination bronchodilator is more effective than individual components. The simplest of these study designs compare a fixed combination of two agents with its individual components. A number of such studies have demonstrated the superiority of a combination of an anticholinergic and a beta agonist to the drugs individually (see below). Such studies, however, have been critiqued on the basis of dose ranging (35–41); that is, the most conventionally used doses of beta agonists and of anticholinergics result in submaximal bronchodilatation. If the dose of an individual agent is increased, some studies appear to show that ''maximal'' bronchodilatation can be achieved. Further improvements in airflow cannot be accomplished either with further increase in the dose of the initial agent or by the addition of a second bronchodilator.

Dose-ranging studies of bronchodilators are complicated by several factors including their method of administration. While bronchodilators can be given effectively by systemic routes, the preferred route of administration is by inhalation. Inhalation can result in the deposition of relatively large amounts in the airway with much smaller systemic absorption. As a result, systemic side effects can be minimized while maintaining effective local bronchodilation. The delivery of inhaled medications, however, depends on the adequate distribution of ventilation. In patients with COPD, ventilation is notoriously inhomogeneous (4). As a result, there can be substantial differences in the dose deposited to various regions within the lower respiratory tract. This inhomogeneity, therefore, can confound interpretation of dose ranging studies.

Dose-ranging studies designed to find the maximal dose of bronchodilator in a given patient are also confounded by day-to-day variability. That is, the response to a bronchodilator in a given patient can vary from one patient to the next (6,30). This may be due to several different mechanisms, including variations in endogenous cholinergic tone, or to variations in inhomogeneity of the distribution of ventilation. This variability, however, confounds studies comparing multiple doses of different drugs which are often performed in a crossover design on different days.

Assessments of bronchodilator effect are also limited by the physiologic measures used to assess benefits. Certainly the FEV_1 is the most important and most commonly used measure of expiratory airflow. On the other hand, the FEV_1 correlates relatively poorly with symptoms, particularly with dyspnea in patients with established moderately severe COPD (42,43). It appears that inspiratory events may be particularly important in causing subjective symptoms such as dyspnea (44). In this regard, other measures, such as lung volumes (45), including functional residual capacity (FRC) and inspiratory capacity (IC), may be particularly important (46). The effects of exercise on lung function, particularly the effects that lead to dynamic hyperinflation, which increases the work of breathing, may also be particularly important (47). Because combination therapies may affect various physiologic parameters differently, it is important not to make any single physiologic measure the definition of clinical response, but rather to regard it as a surrogate measure.

The effect of bronchodilators on airflow is usually assessed following the acute administration of the agent. The long-term and short-term effects of bronchodilators, however, may not be the same. In one analysis of seven trials conducted for 90 days, short-acting beta-agonists and the anticholinergic ipratropium were both found to be effective bronchodilators at the beginning of the trial (11). After 90 days, the β-agonists were still effective bronchodilators but were less effective, suggesting that some tachyphylaxis had occurred. The anticholinergic had no loss of effectiveness over time. Interestingly, the chronic use of anticholinergic was associated with an improvement in the prebronchodilator lung function, an effect also observed in the lung health study

(8). The improved prebronchodilator lung function with ipratropium was not associated with a change in the progressive decline in lung function, however (8). Beta agonists have not been assessed for an effect on decline of lung function. Nevertheless, differential long-term effects may represent another advantage for combination therapy.

B. Effectiveness

A large number of studies have been reported in varying detail evaluating the effectiveness of combination bronchodilator therapy in patients with COPD. Many of these studies have assessed anticholinergics as one component of the combination (Table 1). While some studies appeared to show an advantage of combination therapy, other studies appear to show no advantage. There are a number of reasons why this discrepancy may exist in the literature. Many of the studies involve relatively small numbers of subjects. As a result, they may have been underpowered to detect differences between combination therapy and component therapy; that is, without fail, studies demonstrate that both combination therapy and single-component therapy result in improved airflow. Because the difference between the effect of combined therapy and individual component therapy is less than the difference between single-component therapy and placebo, a larger number of study subjects are required to demonstrate a statistically significant difference. Thus, while many studies show no difference between combination therapy and single-component therapy, this does not mean that no difference exists. It means merely that no difference was demonstrated in that specific study.

Statistical considerations notwithstanding, several generalizations can be made regarding combination bronchodilator therapy in COPD. First, trials using conventional clinical dosages tend to demonstrate added benefit of combination therapy. Improved magnitude of response, improved duration of response, and both are reported in various studies. Improved airflow with a combination of anticholinergics and beta agonists is observed with a number of different combinations. This suggests that the benefits observed are pharmacologic and due to the class of agent action rather than to a specific effect of a single agent within a class. Finally, benefits of combination therapy have been demonstrated when agents have been administered either through metered dose inhaler or as nebulized solutions. This suggests that benefit is independent of mode of administration, and again supports a true pharmacologic benefit of the combination.

A more difficult question is whether "maximal" bronchodilatation can be achieved with a single agent. To evaluate this question, a number of studies

Table 1 Anticholinergics in Combination Bronchodilator Therapy in COPD

Author	Year	Number	Antichol.	Dose	β-Agonist	Dose	Order	Combo better	Ref.
Addis	79	12	ipra	40 μg	fen	100 μg	seq	trend	72
Barros	84	296	ipra	?	alb	?	seq	yes	73
Brown	84	20	ipra	0.5 mg	alb	5 mg	sim	yes	74
Brown	84	20	ipra	0.5 mg	alb	5 mg	sim	yes	75
Combivent Group	94	534	ipra	40 μg	alb	200 μg	sim	yes	76
Dubole	86	20	ipra	80 μg	fen	200 μg	sim	yes	45
Eston	86	11	ipra	80, 120 μg	alb	200, 800 μg	seq	no	40
Frith	86	24	oxit	200 μg	fen	400 μg	sim	yes	77
Gross	84	10	atr	8 × 0.75 μg	alb	4 × 180 μg	seq	no	28
Guttersohn	75	12[a]	ipra	range	fen	range	seq	at subthreshold	78
Howarth	82	12	ipra	1 mg	alb	5 mg	sim	trend	79
Huhti	86	12	ipra	80 μg	fen	200 μg	sim	yes	80
Ikeda	95	20	ipra	range	alb	5 mg	seq	no	41
Ikeda	95	20	oxit	range	alb	5 mg	seq	no	41
Ikeda	95	20	flu	range	alb	5 mg	seq	no	41
Ikeda	95	24	ipra	40, 80 μg	alb	200, 400 μg	sim	yes	48
Kaik	75	40	ipra	80 μg	fen	400 μg	seq	yes	81
Karpel	90	32	ipra	54 μg	meta	1.95 mg	seq	no	35
Karpel	91	30	ipra	54 μg	meta	1.95 mg	seq	no	36
Karpel	94	48	ipra	40 μg	alb (+theo)	200 μg	sim	yes	82
Krivoy	87	9	ipra	20 μg	terb	250 μg	sim	yes	56
LeDoux	89	12	ipra	40, 80 μg	meta	1.3 mg	seq	no	39
Lees	80	35	ipra	80 μg	alb	400 μg	sim	yes	83

Study									
Lefcoe	82	15	ipra	40 μg	fen + theo	5 mg	sim	yes	84
Leitch	78	24	ipra	40 μg	alb	200 μg	sim	trend	58
Levin	96	195	ipra	250 μg	alb	500 μg	sim	yes	85
Lightbody	78	10	ipra	40 μg	alb	200 μg	sim	yes	86
Lioberes	88	13	ipra	range	alb	range	seq	no	37
Marlin	79	8	ipra	40 μg	fen	400 μg	seq	yes	87
Marlin	79	8	ipra	0.5 mg	fen	2 mg	seq	yes	87
Matera	96	12	ipra	40 μg	salmeterol	50 μg	sim	no	88
Molkenboer	87	27	ipra	40 μg	fen	100 μg	sim	yes	89
Newnham	93	29	ipra	40, 200 μg	terb	500, 5000 μg	seq	no	38
Nossen	87	15	ipra	40 μg	fen	100 μg	sim	yes	55
Patrick	90	50[a]	ipra	80 μg	alb	?	repeated	no	67
Petrie	75	8	ipra	40 μg	alb	200 μg	sim	yes	90
Poppius	73	20	ipra	40 μg	isopren	200 μg	seq	yes	91
Poppius	75	21	ipra	80 μg	isopren	300 μg	seq	no	92
Rebuck	87	51	ipra	.5 mg	fen	1.25 mg	sim	no	66
Serra	86	9	ipra	40–640 μg	fen	100–1600 μg	sim	yes	49
Shrestha	91	55	ipra	65 μg	isoeth	5 mg	seq	yes	93
Starke	82	22	atr	range	alb	range	sim	trend	94
Tang	84	24[a]	ipra	80 μg	fen	200 μg	sim	yes	95
Tashkin	96	213	ipra	500 μg	meta	15 mg	sim	yes	96
Ullah	81	29[a]	ipra	80 μg	alb	400 μg	seq	yes	97
Wessling	92	22	ipra	40, 80 μg	fen	400, 800 μg	sim, seq	yes	98

[a]Inclusion of patients with asthma.
Abbreviations: ipra, ipratropium; oxit, oxitropium; atr, atropine; flu, flutropium; fen, fenoterol; alb, albuterol; meta, metaproterenol; theo, theophylline; tero, terbutaline; isopren, isoprenaline; isoeth, isoetharine; sim, simultaneous; seq, sequential.

have attempted to give increasing doses of a single agent until bronchodilatation reaches a maximal value (37–41). After achieving that value, a bronchodilator of a different class is then added. Studies failing to show a benefit of combination therapy are most often of this design. On the other hand, some studies utilizing this design have demonstrated a benefit of combination (48).

Such studies, however, are difficult to interpret. First of all, achieving maximal bronchodilatation may be difficult and may require extraordinarily high doses of conventionally used bronchodilators. Thus, many of the studies may not have achieved maximal bronchodilatation with the doses used. Second, administering drugs sequentially raises the possibility that pharmacokinetic effects could be superimposed on the observations made. Finally, the responses of individual patients are quite variable. Thus, maximal bronchodilatation on one day may not be equivalent to maximal bronchodilatation on another day. An ideal study to evaluate this question, therefore, would evaluate single administration of varying doses of bronchodilators including very high doses on different days with multiple days of testing for each dose. A dose-ranging study using increasing doses of each component and each combination on separate days has shown a benefit of combination over the entire range (49). Thus, the issue of whether a single agent can achieve maximal bronchodilatation remains unresolved. Nevertheless, certain conclusions can be drawn from the available data.

Combinations of anticholinergic bronchodilators together with beta-agonist bronchodilators appear to be more effective than single agents over the dose range most likely to be used clinically. There also appears to be considerable variation in response from patient to patient. Thus, the appropriate use of bronchodilators in an individual patient is likely to require empirical evaluation. A reasonable guideline for clinical use, therefore, would be to use a single bronchodilator agent. If this does not result in sufficient improvement, even at high doses, it is entirely reasonable to add a second agent. The availability of combined β-agonist and anticholinergic agents within a single metered dose inhaler greatly simplifies such therapy.

Such combinations are well received by patients (50,51). The use of fixed combinations decreases the ability of the clinician to titrate the relative doses of the components in an individual patient. On the other hand, it can greatly simplify a drug regimen and can improve patient adherence with a drug regimen. Finally, theophylline can be added to a regimen if the combination of β-agonist and anticholinergic is incompletely satisfactory. As noted above, combination of theophylline with β-agonists results in increased bronchodilatation. The combination of theophylline with anticholinergic has also been noted to cause an increase in airflow beyond that of a single drug (52). Perhaps most importantly, theophylline can be added to the combination of an anticholinergic and a β-agonist and result in further improvement (53,54). Withdrawal of theophylline results in symptomatic decline (13).

Use of a combined therapy is likely to have several benefits. First, there may be a greater magnitude of effect. Second, combined therapy is likely to have less toxicity for a given degree of effect than a high dose of a single bronchodilator, as most toxicities are dose-related. Since beta agonists and anticholinergics have quite different toxicities, this may have considerable clinical practicality. Third, as noted above, most clinical trials have evaluated airflow as the FEV_1. On the other hand, changes in lung volumes (55), changes related to inspiratory efforts (44), and changes in dynamic hyperinflation (56,57), all of which may be related to each other, may be particularly important in affecting subjective perception of dyspnea. Benefits in such parameters have not been as thoroughly studied as changes in FEV_1, but appear to be at least as amenable to improvement with combination therapy if not more so. Improvements in exercise performance (57–62), ventilation perfusion matching (63), and sleep (64) may occur with bronchodilator therapy independent of changes in FEV_1. Thus, even with a modest improvement in lung function as measured by FEV_1, subjective responses to combination treatment should be closely monitored, as other benefits are possible.

Combination therapy with an anticholinergic and a beta agonist has been less extensively evaluated in asthma than in COPD (65–71). Nevertheless, the rationale for the use of combined drug treatment and the issues are similar. Since a single agent can frequently completely reverse the airflow limitation in asthma, combined therapy is less often needed than in COPD, where airflow limitation is always present. Nevertheless in patients with severe disease whose lung function is very often significantly impaired, in individuals who experience dose-related toxicity to β-agonist, and in individuals with severe acute exacerbations, addition of an anticholinergic can be considered. Benefits of such combined therapy have been reported, although this remains a controversial area.

IV. Conclusion

Most patients with symptomatic chronic obstructive pulmonary disease will require long-term bronchodilator therapy. Some patients may receive adequate benefit from a single drug. In many patients, however, the response to a single agent will not be satisfactory. For these individuals, combination therapy with a beta agonist combined with an anticholinergic is reasonable. Theophylline can be added to such a combination with some expectation of added benefit. Advantages of combination therapy include reduced dose of individual components and, hence, less toxicity, improved pharmacodynamics of the combination over individual components, and, possibly, reduced tachyphylaxis. Finally, it is likely that currently used "bronchodilator" therapy has clinical benefits independent of FEV_1. Combination therapy may also be beneficial through such effects. As a result, many patients with symptomatic chronic obstructive pulmonary disease are on combination therapy. The availability of fixed combination devices, while decreasing flexibility for dosing, will certainly improve compliance with regimens depending on multiple medications.

References

1. Stephens NL, Wang J, Halayko AJ. Airway smooth muscle contraction. In: Barnes PJ, Grunstein MM, Leff AR, Woolcock AJ, eds. Asthma. Philadelphia: Lippincott-Raven, 1997:759–800.
2. Persson CGA. Plasma exudation. In: Barnes PJ, Grunstein MM, Leff AR, Woolcock AJ, eds. Asthma. Philadelphia: Lippincott-Raven, 1997:917–924.
3. Tavakoli S, Levine SJ, Shelhamer JH. Airway mucus secretion. In: Barnes PJ, Grunstein MM, Leff AR, Woolcock AJ, eds. Asthma. Philadelphia: Lippincott-Raven, 1997:843–857.
4. Niewoehner DE. Anatomic and pathophysiological correlations in COPD. In: Baum GL, Crapo JD, Celli BR, Karlinsky JB, eds. Textbrook of Pulmonary Diseases. Philadelphia: Lippincott-Raven, 1998:823–842.
5. Barnes PJ. Airway pharmacology. In: Murray JF, Nadel JA, eds. Textbook of Respiratory Medicine. Philadelphia: W.B. Saunders, 1994:1:285–311.
6. Anthonisen NR, Wright E, Group IT. Bronchodilator response in chronic obstructive pulmonary disease. Am Rev Respir Dis 1986; 133:814–819.
7. Nisar M, Walshaw M, Earis JE, Pearson MG, Calverley PMA. Assessment of reversibility of airway obstruction in patients with chronic obstructive airways disease. Thorax 1990; 45:190–194.
8. Anthonisen NR, Connett JE, Kiley JP, et al. Effects of smoking intervention and the use of an inhaled anticholinergic bronchodilator on the rate of decline of FEV_1. JAMA 1994; 272:1497–1505.
9. Braun SR, Levy SF. Comparison of ipratropium bromide and albuterol in chronic obstructive pulmonary disease: a three-center study. Am J Med 1991; 91:28S–32S.
10. Tashkin DP, Ashutosh K, Bleecker ER, et al. Comparison of the anticholinergic bronchodilator ipratropium bromide with metaproterenol in chronic obstructive pulmonary disease. Am J Med 1986; 81:81–89.
11. Rennard SI, Serby CW, Ghafouri M, Johnson PA, Friedman M. Extended therapy

with ipratropium is associated with improved lung function in COPD: a retrospective analysis of data from seven clinical trials. Chest 1996; 110:62–70.
12. Rabe KF, Dent G. Theophylline. In: Barnes PJ, Grunstein MM, Leff AR, Woolcock AJ, eds. Asthma. Philadelphia: Lippincott-Raven, 1997:1535–1554.
13. Kirsten DK, Wegner RE, Jorres RA, Magnussen H. Effects of theophylline withdrawal in severe chronic obstructive pulmonary disease. Chest 1993; 104:1101–1107.
14. Thomas P, Pugsley JA, Stewart JH. Theophylline and salbutamol improve pulmonary function in patients with irreversible chronic obstructive pulmonary disease. Chest 1992; 101:160–165.
15. Dullinger D, Kronenberg R, Niewoehner DE. Efficacy of inhaled metaproterenol and orally-administered theophylline in patients with chronic airflow obstruction. Chest 1986; 89:171–173.
16. Jenne JW. Theophylline as a bronchodilator in COPD and its combination with inhaled β-adrenergic drugs. Chest 1987; 92:7S–14S.
17. Tandon MK, Kailis SG. Bronchodilator treatment for partially reversible chronic obstructive airways disease. Thorax 1991; 46:248–251.
18. Mahler DA. Sustained-released theophylline reduces dyspnea in nonreversible obstructive airway disease. Am Rev Respir Dis 1985; 131:22–25.
19. Filuk RB, Easton PA, Anthonisen NR. Responses to large doses of salbutamol and theophylline in patients with chronic obstructive pulmonary disease. Am Rev Respir Dis 1985; 132:871–874.
20. Lamont H, Van der Straeten M, Pauwels R, Moerman E, Bogaert M. The combined effect of theophylline and terbutaline in patients with chronic obstructive airway diseases. Eur J Respir Dis 1982; 63:13–22.
21. Taylor DR, Buick B, Kinney C, Lowry RC, McDevitt DG. The efficacy of orally administered theophylline, inhaled salbutamol, and a combination of the two as chronic therapy in the management of chronic bronchitis with reversible air-flow obstruction. Am Rev Respir Dis 1985; 131:747–751.
22. Aubier M. Effect of theophylline on diaphragmatic muscle function. Chest 1987; 92:27S–31S.
23. Wanner A. Effects of methylxanthines on airway mucociliary function. Am J Med 1985; 79:16–21.
24. Pasteline G, Mendez R, Kabela E, Farah A. The search for a digitalis substitute II milrinone (Win 47203). Its action on the heart-lung preparation of the dog. Life Sci 1983; 33:1787–1796.
25. Douglas NJ, Davidson I, Sudlow MF, Flenley DC. Bronchodilatation and the site of airway resistance in severe chronic bronchitis. Thorax 1979; 34:51–56.
26. Gross NJ, Petty TL, Friedman M, Skorodin MS, Silvers GW, Donohue JF. Dose response to ipratropium as a nebulized solution in patients with chronic obstructive pulmonary disease. Am Rev Respir Dis 1989; 139:1188–1191.
27. Nisar M, Earis JE, Pearson MG, Calverley PMA. Acute bronchodilator trials in chronic obstructive pulmonary disease. Am Rev Respir Dis 1992; 146:555–559.

28. Gross NJ, Skorodin MS. Role of the parasympathetic system in airway obstruction due to emphysema. N Engl J Med 1984; 311:421–425.
29. Braun S. A comparison of the effect of ipratropium and albuterol in the treatment of chronic obstructive airway disease. Arch Intern Med 1989; 149:544–547.
30. Jaeschke R, Guyatt GH, Cook D, et al. The effect of increasing doses of β-agonists on airflow in patients with chronic airflow limitation. Respir Med 1993; 87:433–438.
31. Levy SF. Bronchodilators in COPD. Chest 1991; 99:793–794.
32. Barnes PJ, Basbaum CB, Nadel JA. Autoradiographic localization of autonomic receptors in airway smooth muscle. Marked differences between large and small airways. Am Rev Respir Dis 1983; 127:758–762.
33. Hoffman EA, Chiplunkar R, Casale TB. CT scanning confirms beta receptor distribution is greater for smaller vs. larger airways. Am J Respir Crit Care Med 1997; 155:A855.
34. Celli BR, Snider GL, Heffner J, et al. Standards for the diagnosis and care of patients with chronic obstructive pulmonary disease. Am J Respir Crit Care Med 1995; 152:S77–S120.
35. Karpel JP, Pesin J, Greenberg D, Gentry E. A comparison of the effects of ipratropium bromide and metaproterenol sulfate in acute exacerbations of COPD. Chest 1990; 98:835–839.
36. Karpel JP. Bronchodilator responses to anticholinergic and beta-adrenergic agents in acute and stable COPD. Chest 1991; 99:871–876.
37. Lloberes P, Ramis L, Montserrat JM, et al. Effect of three different bronchodilators during an exacerbation of chronic obstructive pulmonary disease. Eur Respir J 1988; 1:536–539.
38. Newnham DM, Dhillon DP, Winter JH, Jackson CM, Clark RA, Lipworth BJ. Bronchodilator reversibility to low and high doses of terbutaline and ipratropium bromide in patients with chronic obstructive pulmonary disease. Thorax 1995; 48:1151–1155.
39. LeDoux EJ, Morris JF, Temple WP, Duncan C. Standard and double dose ipratropium bromide and combined ipratropium bromide and inhaled metaproterenol in COPD. Chest 1989; 95:1013–1016.
40. Easton PA, Jadue C, Dhingra S, Anthonisen NR. A comparison of the bronchodilating effects of a beta-2 adrenergic agent (albuterol) and an anticholinergic agent (ipratropium bromide), given by aerosol alone or in sequence. N Engl J Med 1986; 315:735–739.
41. Ikeda A, Nishimura K, Koyama H, Izumi T. Comparative dose-response study of three anticholinergic agents and fenoterol using a metered dose inhaler in patients with chronic obstructive pulmonary disease. Thorax 1995; 50:62–66.
42. O'Donnell DE, Bertley JC, Chau LK, Webb KA. Qualitative aspects of exertional breathlessness in chronic airflow limitation. Am J Respir Crit Care Med 1997; 1555:109–115.
43. Maltais F, Reissmann H, Gottfried SB. Pressure support reduces inspiratory ef-

fort and dyspnea during exercise in chronic airflow obstruction. Am J Respir Crit Care Med 1995; 151:1027–1033.
44. Gorini M, Misuri G, Corrado A, et al. Breathing pattern and carbon dioxide retention in severe chronic obstructive pulmonary disease. Thorax 1996; 51:677–683.
45. Dubois PEP, Delwiche JP, Minette P, Lulling J, Prignot J. Bronchodilating and density dependence effects of fenoterol, ipratropium bromide and duovent in reversible chronic obstructive pulmonary disease. Respiration 1986; 50:280–284.
46. Yan S, Kaminski D, Sliwinski P. Reliability of inspiratory capacity for estimating end-expiratory lung volume changes during exercise in patients with chronic obstructive pulmonary disease. Am J Respir Crit Care Med 1997; 156:55–59.
47. Gibson GJ. Pulmonary hyperinflation a clinical overview. Eur Respir J 1996; 9:2640–2649.
48. Ikeda A, Nishimura K, Koyama H, Izumi T. Bronchodilating effects of combined therapy with clinical dosages of ipratropium bromide and salbutamol for stable COPD: comparison with ipratropium bromide alone. Chest 1995; 107:401–405.
49. Serra C, Giacopelli A, Luciani G. Acute controlled study of the dose-response relationship of fenoterol, ipratropium bromide and their combination. Respiration 1986; 50:144–147.
50. Rammeloo RHU, Luursema PB, Sips AP, Beumer HM, Wald FDM, Cornelissen PJG. Therapeutic equivalence of a fenoterol–ipratropium bromide combination (Berodual) inhaled as a dry powder and by metered dose inhaler in chronic obstructive airway disease. Respiration 1992; 59:322–326.
51. Morton O. Response to duovent of chronic reversible airways obstruction—a controlled trial in general practice. Postgrad Med J 1984; 60:32–35.
52. Bleecker ER, Britt EJ. Acute bronchodilating effects of ipratropium bromide and theophylline in chronic obstructive pulmonary disease. Am J Med 1991; 91:24S–27S.
53. Nishimura K, Koyama H, Ikeda A, Izumi T. Is oral theophylline effective in combination with both inhaled anticholinergic agent and inhaled beta$_2$-agonist in the treatment of stable COPD? Chest 1993; 104:179–184.
54. Nishimura K, Koyama H, Ikeda A, Sugiura N, Kawakatsu K, Izumi T. The additive effect of theophylline on a high-dose combination of inhaled salbutamol and ipratropium bromide in stable COPD. Chest 1995; 107:718–723.
55. Nossen GD, Van de Mark T, Postma DS, Koeter GH, Peset R, De Zeeuw RA. Berodual versus its single components fenoterol and ipratropium bromide. A placebo controlled trial in chronic bronchitis. Postgrad Med J 1987; 63:19a.
56. Krivoy N, Jubarin A, Gaitini L, Rubin A, Alroy G. Combination therapy of ipratropium bromide, terbutaline and slow release theophylline in asthma and chronic airways obstruction. Postgrad Med J 1987; 63:21a.
57. Belman MJ, Botnick WC, Shin JW. Inhaled bronchodilators reduce dynamic hyperinflation during exercise in patients with chronic obstructive pulmonary disease. Am J Respir Crit Care Med 1996; 153:967–975.

58. Leitch AG, Hopkin JM, Ellis DA, Merchant S, McHardy GJR. The effect of aerosol ipratropium bromide and salbutamol on exercise tolerance in chronic bronchitis. Thorax 1978; 33:711–713.
59. Berger R, Smith D. Effect of inhaled metaproterenol on exercise performance in patients with stable "fixed" airway obstruction. Am Rev Respir Dis 1988; 138:624–629.
60. Ikeda A, Nishimura K, Koyama H, Tsukino M, Mishima M, Izumi T. Dose response study of ipratropium bromide aerosol on maximum exercise performance in stable patients with chronic obstructive pulmonary disease. Thorax 1996; 51:48–53.
61. Fink G, Kaye C, Sulkes J, Gabbay U, Spitzer SA. Effect of theophylline on exercise performance in patients with severe chronic obstructive pulmonary disease. Thorax 1994; 49:332–334.
62. Leitch AG, Morgan A, Ellis DA, Bell G, Haslett C, McHardy GJR. Effect of oral salbutamol and slow-release aminophylline on exercise tolerance in chronic bronchitis. Thorax 1981; 36:787–789.
63. Ashutosh K, Dev G, Steele D. Nonbronchodilator effects of pirbuterol and ipratropium in chronic obstructive pulmonary disease. Chest 1995; 107:173–178.
64. Berry RB, Desa MM, Branum JP, Light RW. Effect of theophylline on sleep and sleep-disordered breathing in patients with chronic obstructive pulmonary disease. Am Rev Respir Dis 1991; 142:245–250.
65. Wolfe JD, Tashkin DP, Calvarese B, Simmons M. Bronchodilator effects of terbutaline and aminophylline alone and in combination in asthmatic patients. N Engl J Med 1978; 298:363–367.
66. Rebuck AS, Chapman KR. Nebulized anticholinergic and sympathomimetic treatment of asthma and chronic obstructive airways disease in the emergency room. Am J Med 1987; 82:59–64.
67. Patrick DM, Dales RE, Stark RM, Laliberte G, Dickinson G. Severe exacerbations of COPD and asthma. Chest 1990; 98:295–297.
68. Ward MJ, Macfarlane JT, Davies D. A place for ipratropium bromide in the treatment of severe acute asthma. Br J Dis Chest 1985; 79:374–378.
69. Ward MJ, Fentem PH, Smith WHR, Davies D. Ipratropium bromide in acute asthma. BMJ 1981; 282:598–602.
70. Ruffin RE, Fitzgerald JD, Rebuck AS. A comparison of the bronchodilator activity of Sch 1000 and salbutamol. J Allergy Clin Immunol 1977; 59:136–141.
71. Boushey HA. Combination therapy with anticholinergic agents for airflow obstruction. Postgrad Med J 1987; 63:69–74.
72. Addis GJ, Barclay J, Chang EM. Assessment of a combination of doses of fenoterol and ipratropoium suitable for a single metered-dose aerosol. Eur J Clin Pharmacol 1979; 16:97–100.
73. Barros MJ, Rees PJ. Bronchodilator responses to salbutamol followed by ipratropium bromide in partially reversible airflow obstruction. Respir Med 1990; 84:371–375.
74. Brown JG, Chan CS, Kelly CA, Dent AG, Zimmerman PV. Assessment of the

clinical usefulness of nebulised ipratropium bromide in patients with chronic airflow limitation. Thorax 1984; 39:272–276.
75. Brown IG, Chan CS, Kelly CA, Dent AG, Zimmerman PV. Assessment of the clinical usefulness of nebulised ipratropium bromide in patients with chronic airflow limitation. Thorax 1984; 39:272–276.
76. Combivent Inhalational Aerosol Study Group. In chronic obstructive pulmonary disease, a combination of ipratropium and albuterol is more effective than either agent alone. Chest 1994; 105:1411–1419.
77. Frith PA, Jenner B, Atkinson J. Effects of inhaled oxitropium and fenoterol, alone and in combination, in chronic airflow obstruction. Respiration 1986; 50: 294–297.
78. Gutersohn J, Joos H, Herzog H. The effect of R_{aw} on Sch 1000 MDI or fenoterol MDI and the combined administration of subthreshold dosages of both compounds. Postgrad Med J 1975; 51:113–114.
79. Howarth PH, Stainforth JN, Holgate ST. Bronchodilator efficacy of nebulised salbutamol and ipratropium bromide in chronic airflow obstruction. Thorax 1982; 37:789.
80. Huhti E, Poukkula A. Comparison of fenoterol, ipratropium bromide and their combination in patients with asthma or chronic airflow obstruction. Respiration 1986; 50:298–301.
81. Kaik G. The effect on total airways resistance (R_t) of adding Sch 1000 MDI to beta-adrenergics, and vice versa, in patients with chronic bronchitis and emphysema. Postgrad Med J 1975; 51:114–115.
82. Karpel JP, Kotch A, Zinny M, Pesin J, Alleyne W. A comparison of inhaled ipratropium, oral theophylline plus inhaled beta-agonist, and the combination of all three in patients with COPD. Chest 1994; 105:1089–1094.
83. Lees AW, Allan GW, Smith J. Nebulised ipratropium bromide and salbutamol in chronic bronchitis. Br J Clin Prac 1980; 34:340–342.
84. Lefcoe NM, Toogood JH, Blennerhassett G, Baskerville J, Paterson NAM. The addition of an aerosol anticholinergic to an oral beta agonist plus theophylline in asthma and bronchitis. Chest 1982; 82:300–305.
85. Levin DC, Little KS, Laughlin KR, et al. Addition of anticholinergic solution prolongs bronchodilator effect of beta 2 agonists in patients with chronic obstructive pulmonary disease. Am J Med 1996; 100:40S–48S.
86. Lightbody IM, Ingram CG, Legge JS, Johnston RN. Ipratropium bromide, salbutamol and predisolone in bronchial asthma and chronic bronchitis. Br J Dis Chest 1978; 72:181–187.
87. Marlin GE, Berend N, Harrison AC. Combined cholinergic antagonist and beta 2-adrenoceptor agonist bronchodilator therapy by inhalation. Aust N Z J Med 1979; 9:511–514.
88. Matera MG, Caputi M, Cazzola M. A combination with clinical recommended dosages of salmeterol and ipratropium is not more effective than salmeterol alone in patients with chronic obstructive pulmonary disease. Respir Med 1996; 90: 497–499.

89. Molkenboer JFWM, Cornelissen PJG. A double-blind randomized crossover study assessing the efficacy of Berodual in comparison to its componennts ipratropium bromide and fenoterol in chronic bronchitis. Postgrad Med J 1987; 63: 19a.
90. Petrie GR, Palmer KNV. Comparison of aerosol ipratropium bromide and salbutamol in chronic bronchitis and asthma. Br Med J 1975; 1:430–432.
91. Poppius H, Salorinne Y. Comparative trial of a new anticholinergic bronchodilator, Sch 1000, and salbutamol in chronic bronchitis. Br Med J 1973; 4:134–136.
92. Poppius H, Salorinne Y, Viljanen AA. Changes in airways resistance (R_{aw}) in asthmatics and bronchitics following Sch 1000 MDI and additional beta-adrenergics. Postgrad Med J 1975; 51:118–119.
93. Shrestha M, O'Brien T, Haddox R, Gourlay HS, Reed G. Decreased duration of emergency department treatment of chronic obstructive pulmonary disease exacerbations with the addition of ipratropium bromide to beta-agonist therapy. Ann Emerg Med 1991; 20:1206–1209.
94. Starke ID, Parker RA, Turner-Warwick M. Atropine methonitrate and salbutamol in chronic airways obstruction: peak effect and duration of action. Respiration 1982; 42:51–56.
95. Tang OT, Flatley M. A comparison of effects on inhaling a combined preparation of fenoterol with ipratropium bromide (Duovent) with those of fenoterol and salbutamol. Postgrad Med J 1984; 60:24–27.
96. Tashkin DP, Bleecker E, Braun S, et al. Results of a multicenter study of nebulized inhalant bronchodilator solution. Am J Med 1996; 100:62S–69S.
97. Ullah M, Newman GB, Saunders KB. Influence of age on response to ipatropium and salbutamol in asthma. Thorax 1981; 36:523–529.
98. Wesseling G, Mostert R, Wouters EFM. A comparison of the effects of anticholinergic and beta-2 agonist and combination therapy on respiratory impedance in COPD. Chest 1992; 101:166–173.

8

Tiotropium (Ba 679)
Pharmacology and Early Clinical Observations

THEODORE J. WITEK, JR.

Boehringer Ingelheim Pharmaceuticals, Inc.
Ridgefield, Connecticut
and Mount Sinai School of Medicine
New York, New York

CHARLES W. SERBY

Boehringer Ingelheim Pharmaceuticals, Inc.
Ridgefield, Connecticut

JOSEPH F. SOUHRADA

Boehringer Ingelheim Pharmaceuticals, Inc.
Ridgefield
and Yale University School of Medicine
New Haven, Connecticut

BERND DISSE

Boehringer Ingelheim
Ingelheim, Germany

I. Introduction

Inhaled antimuscarinic compounds have a long history of respiratory therapeutics ranging from the use of henbane (*Hyoscyamus*) in the Pre-Christian Era to the currently widely prescribed bronchodilator ipratropium bromide (1,2). Development of ipratropium bromide was a clear advance in bronchodilator therapy as its quaternary structure afforded limited absorption, an excellent safety profile, and significant local bronchodilatory activity (3,4). As a class-selective but not subtype-selective muscarinic receptor antagonist, its use over the past three decades has confirmed its safety and efficacy in clinical practice.

The next important milestone in antimuscarinic airway pharmacology came with the discovery of tiotropium bromide and its characterization as a long-acting, specific muscarinic antagonist with a unique mechanism of subtype selectivity (5–8). With this preclinical profile established, clinical development was initiated to confirm its therapeutic potential in patients, particularly those with chronic obstructive pulmonary disease (COPD), where vagal tone may be the principal reversible element of airway obstruction. This chapter will overview the important preclinical observations and describe the early clinical studies supportive of significant potential to provide therapeutic management of the reversible component of bronchoconstriction associated with COPD.

II. Pharmacology

A. Chemistry

The structural formula for tiotropium is illustrated in Figure 1 alongside the congeneer antimuscarinic drugs atropine and ipratropium. Like ipratropium, tiotropium is distinguished from atropine by its positively charged quaternary ammonium structure, which is responsible for the limited gastrointestinal absorption. The thiophene groups on tiotropium add to the molecule's lipophilicity. The compound's very high affinity and slow dissociation (discussed below), however, is not currently explained by chemical structure.

B. Receptor Kinetics

As discussed in detail in Chapter 2, muscarinic receptor subtypes serve different regulatory functions. Importantly, the bronchoconstrictor and mucous se-

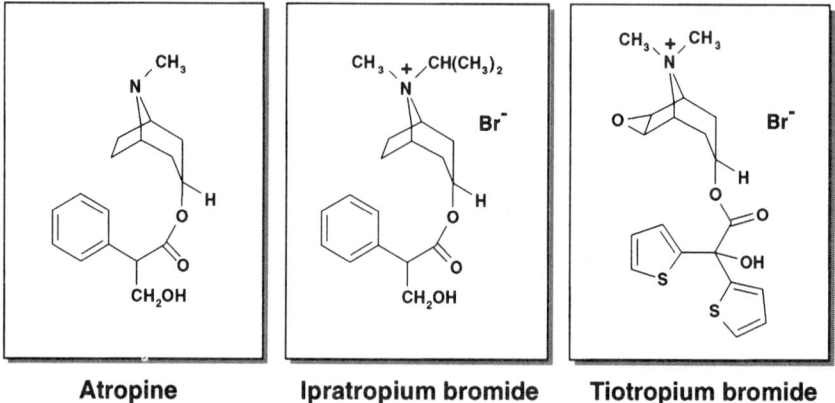

Figure 1 Chemical structures of atropine, ipratropium bromide, and tiotropium bromide.

cretory response to acetylcholine and cholinergic nerve stimulation is postjunctionally mediated primarily through M_3 receptors, while the prejunctional M_2 receptors on postganglionic cholinergic nerves have an autoinhibitory effect on acetylcholine (ACh) release. Following this concept, M_3-subtype selectivity of an inhibitor has pharmacological advantages that may have useful therapeutic implications.

Initial studies comparing the receptor-antagonist dissociation kinetics of tiotropium to other muscarinic antagonists were encouraging (5). Apparent binding affinity (K_D), as demonstrated in Chinese hamster ovary cells transfected with human muscarinic (Hm) receptor subtype cDNA, was generally higher (i.e., lower K_D) for tiotropium than for ipratropium and essentially not different between the muscarinic receptor subtypes. Tiotropium dissociated over 100 times more slowly than ipratropium bromide from the muscarinic receptors. As a unique feature, kinetic selectivity of tiotropium was observed meaning that the compound dissociates much slower from M_1 and M_3 receptors than from the M_2 receptor (Table 1).

In vitro studies with the human lung (7) confirmed tiotropium's high binding affinity and slow dissociation. Tiotropium is about tenfold more potent than atropine and ipratropium bromide in displacing specific [^{3}H]N-methylscopolamine binding.

C. Isolated Airway: Muscle Contraction

Reversible antagonism of methacholine-induced (isotonic) contraction of guinea pig tracheal segments was observed following incubation with tiotropium in concentrations of 6×10^{-10} to 6×10^{-9} M (5). Similar rightward shifts in the concentration response were seen for glycopyrrolate, ipratropium bromide, and atropine; tiotropium (Ba679 BR) was most potent in this assay (Fig. 2).

Table 1 Dissociation Half-Lives of Receptor-Drug Complexes (Half-Life [in hours] ± SD)

	M_1 [h]	M_2 [h]	M_3 [h]
^{3}H-ipratropium iodide	0.11 ± 0.005	0.035 ± 0.005	0.26 ± 0.02
^{3}H-tiotropium iodide	14.6 ± 2.2	3.6 ± 0.5	34.7 ± 2.9

Source: Ref. 5.

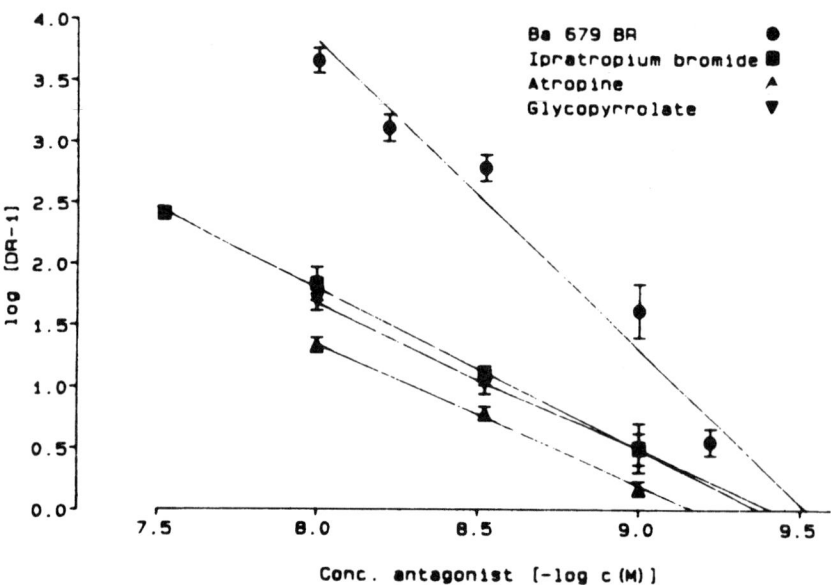

Figure 2 Schild plot: antagonism of antimuscarinic compounds against methacholine-induced contraction of guinea pig tracheal rings in vitro. (From Ref. 5.)

D. Isolated Cells: Ciliary Beat Frequency

Ciliary beat frequency was evaluated in isolated guinea pig ciliated cells maintained in primary culture (5). Following near-maximal stimulation of the beat frequency with methacholine (10^{-5}M), the continuously superfused cells were equilibrated with tiotropium at concentrations known to inhibit methacholine stimulation. The superfusion was then switched from the antagonists to the agonist, and ciliary beat frequency was repeatedly measured. Following ipratropium "washout," stimulation was established at the first measurement point of 16 min while a comparable stimulation of cilia was not seen until 82 min after tiotropium "washout." These observations show that dissociation kinetics of tiotropium controls its long duration of action.

E. Isolated Airway: ACh Release

In guinea pig as well as human trachea, tiotropium and atropine equally enhance electric field–stimulated release of ACh (8), which reflects prejunctional M_2-receptor blockade. This enhancement was lost 2 hours after washout of

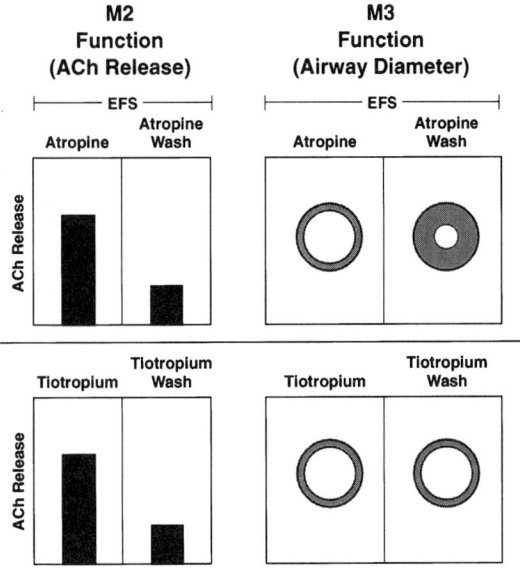

Figure 3 Functional consequence of M_3 receptor selectivity. Enhancement of ACh release with electric field stimulation (EFS) (M_2 function) is lost 2 hours after washout (Wash) of atropine and tiotropium. Inhibition of EFS induced contraction (M_3 function), however, is lost following an atropine washout but not after tiotropium washout. (Data from Ref. 6.)

test drugs, a time when airway smooth muscle contraction, mediated postjunctionally by M_3 receptors, was still blocked by tiotropium but not by atropine. These experiments functionally demonstrate the M_3-receptor selectivity of tiotropium (Fig. 3).

F. In Vivo Animal Pharmacology

Protection against acetylcholine-induced bronchospasm has been evaluated in dogs that were anaesthetized and ventilated (5). Acetylcholine was administered intravenously before and after antimuscarinic agent inhalation with measurement of pulmonary resistance used to determine provocation endpoint. Tiotropium aerosol from a 0.3 g/L solution gave a similar degree of protection as an ipratropium bromide aerosol from a 1.0 g/L solution (Fig. 4). The time course of the maintenance of protection was dose-dependent for both antagonists, with a sustaining of response particularly notable with tiotropium. In the same experiments, neither antagonist affected left ventricular function.

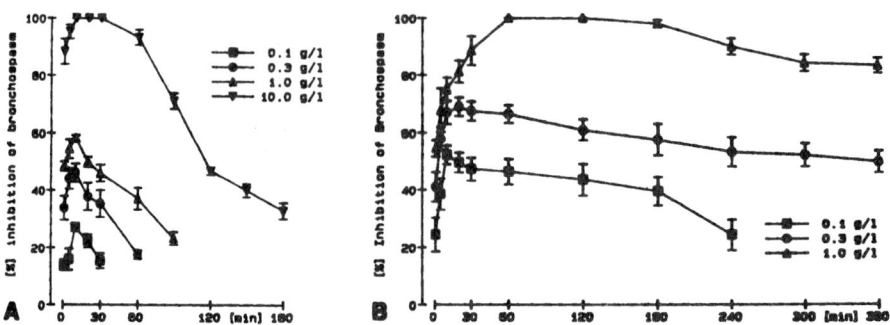

Figure 4 Time course of protection against acetycholine-induced bronchospasms by inhaled (A) ipratropium bromide or (B) tiotropium. Mean ± SEM, n = 6 dogs for each concentration. (From Ref. 5.)

III. Human Pharmacology and Early Clinical Trials

A. Preliminary Human Pharmacokinetics

Several single-dose escalating trials with tiotropium were conducted in normal volunteers. There were no relevant drug-related effects on vital signs (pulse rate and blood pressure), electrocardiography, pupillometry, saliva secretion, or routine laboratory parameters. After inhalation of tiotropium, plasma levels attained a maximum 5 min postdose with subsequent rapid decline (<1 hour) to very low levels in the 3 pg/mL (6pM) range. At this low level plasma tiotropium terminal phase half-life was determined to be 5–6 days, independent of dose. Airway resistance (R_{aw}), as determined by body plethysmography was also analyzed in normal volunteers. After inhalation of tiotropium, a slight decrease in R_{aw} was observed at higher doses. This decrease in R_{aw} lasted 72 hours.

In multiple-dose studies in healthy normal volunteers, minimal adverse events were reported, the majority in higher doses. Similarly, as in single-dose trials there were no relevant drug-related effects on vital signs, electrocardiography, pupillometry, saliva secretion, or routine laboratory parameters.

B. Effects in Asthmatics

One trial that evaluated bronchodilator response and methacholine antagonism in mild asthmatics following tiotropium has been reported (9). This trial allowed for early characterization of bronchodilator response and confirmation of dose and duration of action. This study included 12 patients with mild disease, i.e., documented hyperresponsiveness to inhaled methacholine with a provoking concentration causing a 20% fall in FEV_1 (PC_{20}) of less than 8 mg/mL and near normal baseline pulmonary function. All were atopic as defined by a positive skin response to common allergens. None had suffered an asthma exacerbation nor respiratory infection in the preceding 6 weeks. Each patient had only occasional symptoms, which were controlled by inhaled β-adrenergic agonist therapy alone. The majority of patients had a baseline FEV_1 in excess of 80% of their predicted normal value. Inhaled sympathomimetics and caffeinated beverages were withheld for at least 8 hours before each study.

This study was performed in a randomized double-blind crossover manner consisting of four single-dose treatment periods—placebo, tiotropium 10, 40, and 80 μg. This treatment was administered as a powder in a lactose carrier via a breath-activated inhaler. Because of the long duration of action of tiotropium, each treatment day was separated by a washout period of 8–25 days.

In order to determine a duration of action of tiotropium after a single dose, all patients remained in the hospital for 48 hours to undergo repeated challenges with methacholine at 2, 12, 24, 36, and 48 hours after treatment. Four of the 12 patients also underwent a methacholine challenge 72 hours post-treatment.

Bronchodilation Following Tiotropium

On each study day, tiotropium caused a mild but statistically significant bronchodilation in a time-dependent but not dose-dependent manner (Fig. 5). Bron-

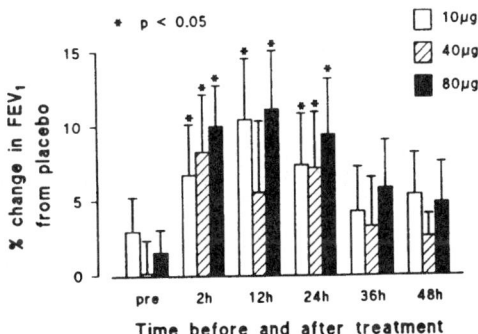

Figure 5 Changes in FEV_1 for each dose of tiotropium compared with placebo, expressed as a percent increase, at each time point before and after treatment (mean ± SEM). (From Ref. 9.)

chodilation was sustained for up to 24 hours and was equivalent for all three doses. The percentage increases for FEV_1 (mean ± SEM) for 10, 40, and 80 µg of tiotropium when compared with placebo at each time point was, respectively, 6.7 ± 3.4, 8.2 ± 3.9, and 10.0 ± 2.7 at 2 h; 10.4 ± 4.1, 5.5 ± 4.8, and 11.1 ± 3.9 at 12 h; 7.3 ± 3.5, 7.1 ± 3.8, and 9.4 ± 3, 7 at 24 h (Fig. 5). At 36 and 48 h after drug administration, airway caliber as evaluated by FEV_1 determinations did not differ significantly from placebo.

Effect of Tiotropium on Methacholine Challenge

Tiotropium provided significant protection against methacholine challenge in all patients (Fig. 6). This protection was sustained for up to 48 hours in a dose- and time-dependent manner. At the 2-hour measurement point, which was the time of peak effect, the protective effect of tiotropium was 5.0 ± 1.1, 7.1 ± 0.5, and 7.9 ± 0.7 doubling doses for 10 µg, 40 µg, and 80 µg, respectively.

Significant protection was seen at all of the other time points for each dose of drug (Fig. 6). At the 36- and 48-hour time points, the protective effect of 10 µg and 40 µg was significantly less than earlier time points for each corresponding dose. At 36 and 48 hours, the 80 µg tiotropium bromide had a greater protective effect than either of the lower doses.

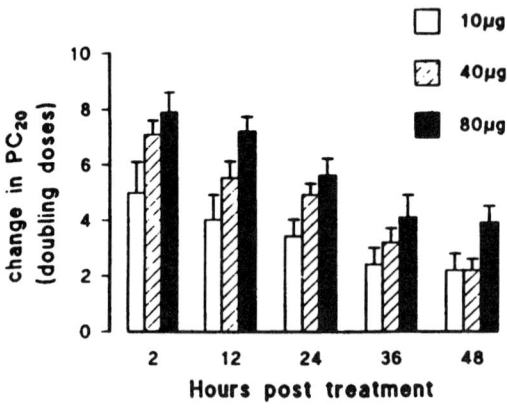

Figure 6 Changes in PC_{20} from placebo for each dose of tiotropium at each time point after treatment, expressed in terms of doubling dose protection (mean ± SEM). (From Ref. 9.)

C. Effects in Patients with COPD

A series of three clinical trials were conducted in patients with COPD in order to characterize the bronchodilator activity of tiotropium. These patients are regarded to have particular therapeutic benefit, given the relatively increased cholinergic component to airflow obstruction (10,11) and the increased submucosal gland secretion (12).

Sequential studies were conducted to evaluate dose and time response of tiotropium. First, a pilot study examined dose ranges of tiotropium bromide from 10 to 160 µg delivered via a piezoelectric driven nebulizer. Next, single doses of 10 to 80 µg tiotropium bromide were evaluated with a lactose powder inhaler. Finally, tiotropium powder in dose ranges of 4.5 to 36 µg were administered over a 28-day period to evaluate dose-response range at steady state. From this last trial on, tiotropium dose labeling utilized the base (e.g., 18 µg tiotropium vs. 20 µg tiotropium bromide) to conform to international dosing conventions.

All patients investigated in the above COPD studies conformed to the American Thoracic Society definition of COPD (13) and were required to meet standard inclusion/exclusion criteria designed to insure exclusion of patients with asthma and other respiratory diseases. Specifically, patients with asthma were not likely to be enrolled because patients were to be older, heavier smokers and to have a medical history void of atopy or allergic rhinitis and have a late onset of respiratory symptoms (Table 2).

Pilot Dose Escalation Study

In this crossover study (14), six patients with moderate COPD (mean baseline FEV_1 was 46% of predicted value) had spirometric and plethysmographic assessments following inhalation of single doses of tiotropium ranging from 9 to 144 µg. Medication was delivered in an aqueous formulation via an ultrasonic nebulizer device.

Table 2 Key Selection Criteria for Patients with Chronic Obstructive Airway Disease

---
Consistent with ATS disease criteria
Aged 40 years or greater
Minimum 10 pack-year smoking history
$FEV_1 < 65\%$ predicted normal
No history of asthma, atopy, allergic rhinitis
Blood eosinophils < 600 mm^3

A general dose order improvement was observed in lung function response, with peak effects observed 90 to 120 min after inhalation. This effect persisted for 12 to 15 hours in most patients with FEV_1, returning to near-predose values at the 19-hour measurement point. An improvement of 20% of FEV_1 from baseline was still apparent 12 hours after dosing with 72 and 144 µg of tiotropium. A "morning dip" in the temporal response was noted at all doses tested that was followed by a spontaneous improvement in response. This presumed circadian variation in cholinergic tone served as the basis for more detailed characterization in the clinical development program.

There were no significant adverse events reported in this small trial. Taken together with the spirometric response, these pilot observations demonstrated the potential of tiotropium as a safe and long-acting bronchodilator for further clinical development in patients with well-defined COPD.

Single-Dose, Dose-Ranging Study

In a second study (15), 35 patients with COPD (mean baseline FEV_1 was equal to 44% of predicted value) were evaluated for spirometric response to single doses of 9 to 72 µg tiotropium. This was a double-blind placebo-controlled crossover study. Medication was delivered as a powder in a lactose carrier via a breath-activated inhaler.

Significant bronchodilation as determined by FEV_1 improvement was confirmed at all doses. Effect was rapid (being observed at the first assessment point of 15 min) with peak effects (19% to 26% of baseline) observed in the range of 1 to 4 hours (Fig. 7). Duration of effect extended to the 32-hour observation period. The morning dip and subsequent recovery of pulmonary function observed in the pilot trial was again noted, with the spontaneous recovery exhibiting a dose-dependent trend.

The relatively large placebo response observed is likely due in part to carryover effects, since the washout time in this study was only 72 hours. If one excludes the patients with significant carryover effect (previous dose >9 µg), the placebo peak response is reduced from 16% to 11%.

The drug was well tolerated at all doses, and no abnormalities were observed in routine laboratory assessments or clinical evaluation. Given these observations, clinical development proceeded to a multiple-dose, dose-ranging study of 1 month's duration.

Multiple-Dose, Dose-Ranging Study

One hundred sixty-nine COPD patients (mean baseline FEV_1 was equal to 42% of predicted value) participated in a randomized, double-blind, placebo-controlled study to evaluate the effect of tiotropium given once daily in doses

Tiotropium (Ba 679)

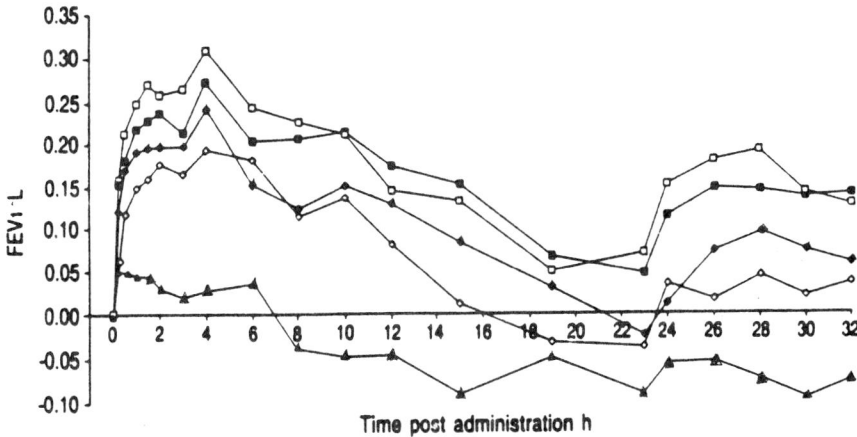

Figure 7 Increase in adjusted mean improvement in FEV_1 from test day baseline, excluding test days which follow tiotropium bromide 20, 40, and 80 µg.–□–: 80 µg tiotropium bromide;–■–: 40 µg tiotropium bromide;–◆–: 20 µg tiotropium bromide; –◇–: 10 µg tiotropium bromide;–▲–: placebo. FEV_1 forced expiratory volume in 1 sec. (From Ref. 15.)

of 4.5, 9.0, 18, or 36 µg for a period of 4 weeks. Study medication was administered by inhalation in the lactose powder formulation. Spirometry was assessed at 0800, 1000, and 1200 hours at weekly visits during baseline (2 weeks), treatment (4 weeks), and posttreatment (3 weeks) periods. During the treatment period, spirometry was also evaluated for 6 hours after dosing.

Preliminary results (16) confirmed the bronchodilating activity of tiotropium over a 1-month treatment period. All doses produced increases in FEV_1 that were significantly greater than placebo at both the start and end of the 24-hour dosing interval. There were no statistically significant differences between doses. Only two serious adverse events were reported, neither considered by the investigator as drug related. No significant changes were observed in routine laboratory parameters and ECGs.

These observations confirmed the bronchodilating activity of tiotropium with repeated treatments and provided the basis for full development in long-term (1 year) clinical trials.

IV. Potential Role in Clinical Practice

With the introduction of ipratropium bromide, antimuscarinic inhalation therapy has gained wide acceptance in the treatment of obstructive airway disease.

As a quaternary compound, its minimal gastrointestinal absorption resulted in a favorable therapeutic window anchored by bronchodilation and minimal systemic effects (11,12). In COPD, ipratropium bromide has emerged as first-line therapy (17) and has a prominent place in treatment standards (13,18). In asthma, the slower onset of action and, in the majority of patients, lower bronchodilating efficacy relative to beta agonists has limited its role in acute relief of bronchospasm. However, some, but not all trials have demonstrated additive effects with beta agonists in acute severe asthma in children (19) and adults (20,21). In rhinitis, ipratropium has been proven effective in reducing the rhinorrhea associated with infection (22,23) and forms of perennial rhinitis (24,25).

The discovery and early development of tiotropium have led the way for a new generation of antimuscarinics suitable for inhalation therapy. Both in vitro and in vivo pharmacology have confirmed its potency, muscarinic receptor selectivity, and extended duration of effect. Early clinical studies have shown excellent tolerability and demonstration of significant bronchodilator effects. There is minimal absorption, and the major portion of the absorbed tiotropium is excreted unchanged in urine. Its apparent lack of metabolism at therapeutic doses will minimize any potential for drug-drug interactions.

Tiotropium's half-life in plasma is approximately 5.5 days. The acute improvement observed in lung function with daily administration lends support to the therapeutically practical once-daily administration. Long-term studies in patients will confirm the safety and efficacy of this dosing interval. This can have meaningful therapeutic benefit in therapy, as patient compliance in COPD has been demonstrated to be suboptimal in long-term trials (26).

As discussed in detail elsewhere in this text, the more rapid "off-kinetics" of tiotropium from M_2 receptors as compared to M_3 and M_1 receptors has theoretical advantages in the treatment of respiratory disease. Whether these kinetic features of tiotropium will translate to in vivo M_3-subtype selectivity and whether this quality is responsible for important features to the practitioner remains to be determined. Pharmacologically, blockade of the M_2 receptor by a nonselective agent can increase ACh release, which can have a countereffect to the desired antagonism of the M_3 receptors on airway smooth muscle and glands. In asthma, there is evidence of dysfunctional M_2 receptors (27–29), which would minimize the importance of receptor-selective antagonists. In COPD, however, the availability of antagonists that avoid or minimize M_2 blockade may possess relatively more advantages over nonselective agents. Although these theoretical advantages of tiotropium are not easily addressed directly in clinical investigation, it is important to note that data at present in both asthma and COPD show tiotropium to be safe, effective, and well tolerated.

Initial observations in patients with COPD are encouraging (14–16). Bronchodilation is observed following single-dose administration, and preliminary observations over 1 month indicate maintained bronchodilation relative to placebo. Although the initial studies focused on standard spirometric variables, it is plausible that prolonged reduction in trapped air volume can translate to decreased sensation of dyspnea and consequent improved exercise performance (30,31). This hypothesis is being evaluated at present. The role in the parasympathetic pathway in altered sleep architecture in COPD patients (32) lends itself to potential therapy of tiotropium in COPD patients with compromised sleep quality. In COPD, hypoventilation along with both increased functional residual capacity (FRC) and altered ventilation/perfusion mismatching contribute to hypoxemia and oxygen desaturation (33). Following treatment with ipratropium, sleep quality and oxygen saturation of patients with COPD was significantly improved (32) but data with tiotropium are not yet available.

Studies with first-generation quarternary antimuscarinics have shown a superior safety profile relative to beta agonists, particularly with respect to cardiovascular side effects (34–36). Additionally, antimuscarinics are void of the ventilation-perfusion abnormality (37) frequently seen with sympathomimetics. Therefore, tiotropium's prolonged duration of action, coupled with unwanted effects of beta agonists on gas exchange, make tiotropium an attractive therapeutic agent for maintenance therapy, including nocturnal morbidity in COPD patients.

Studies to date in asthma have been limited to the report on its bronchodilation and competitive antagonism of methacholine. The magnitude and duration of bronchodilation in a group of relatively mild asthmatics were encouraging. Full clinical characterization of tiotropium have to confirm its clinical potency in asthma. As worsening of asthma during the night is quite common and thought to be due to increased cholinergic tone during sleep (38), the potential for therapeutic benefit exists. Here, once again, single-dose covering the night can have desirable therapeutic benefits. Finally, the relative safety of antimuscarinics over beta agonists give yet further meaningful choices when long-acting bronchodilators are indicated in stepwise asthma management.

V. Summary and Conclusions

Tiotropium has been pharmacologically classified as a long-acting, muscarinic-receptor–specific antagonist, giving it potential for a new generation of bronchodilators. In initial clinical testing, the drug was shown to be safe and well tolerated. Preliminary observations in patients with both asthma and COPD confirm its long-acting bronchodilator properties. In the latter group, testing over a 1-month period confirmed its potential to provide maintenance bronchodilation with once daily dosing. Long-term trials and special studies will help determine its ultimate role in clinical practice and provide the evidence to place this new-generation agent into the therapeutic armamentarium for obstructive airway disease.

References

1. Gandevia B. Historical review of the use of parasympatholytic agents in the treatment of respiratory disorders. Postgraduate Medical Journal 1975; 51:13–20.
2. Chapman KR. History of anticholinergic treatment in airways disease. In: Gross NJ, ed. Anticholinergic therapy in obstructive airways disease. London: Franklin Scientific Publications, 1993:9–17.
3. Gross NJ. Ipratropium bromide. N Engl J Med 1988; 319:486–494.
4. Witek TJ, Schachter EN. Respiratory Care Pharmacology and therapeutics. Philadelphia: W.B. Saunders, 1994.
5. Disse B, Reichl R, Speck G, Traunecker W, Rominger KL, Hammer R. Ba679 BR, a novel anticholinergic bronchodilator. Life Sci 1993; 52:537–544.
6. Barnes PJ, Belvisi MG, Mak JCW, Haddad E, O'Connor B. Tiotropium bromide (Ba 679 BR), a novel long-acting muscarinic antagonist for the treatment of obstructive airways disease. Life Sci 1995; 56:853–859.
7. Haddad E, Mak JCW, Barnes PJ. Characterization of [^{3}H]BA 679. a slow-dissociating muscarinic receptor antagonist in human lung: radioligand binding and autoradiographic mapping. Mol Pharmacol 1994; 45:899–907.
8. Takahaski T, Belvisi MG, Patel H, Ward JK, Tadjkarimi S, Yocub MH, Barnes PJ. Effect of BA679 BR, a novel long-acting anticholinergic agent, on cholinergic neurotransmission in guinea pig and human airways. Am J Respir Crit Care Med 1994; 150:1640–1645.
9. O'Connor BJ, Towse LJ, Barnes PJ. Prolonged effect of tiotropium bromide on methacholine-induced bronchoconstriction in asthma. Am J Respir Crit Care Med 1996; 154:876–880.
10. Barnes PJ. Neural control of human airways in health and disease. Am Rev Respir Dis 1986; 134:1289–1314.
11. Chapman KR. The role of anticholinergic bronchodilators in adult asthma and COPD. Lung 1990; 168:295–303.
12. Gross NJ, Skorodin MS. Anticholinergic, antimuscarinic bronchodilators. Am Rev Respir Dis 1984; 129:856–870.
13. American Thoracic Society. Standards for the diagnosis and care of patients with

chronic obstructive pulmonary disease (COPD) and asthma. Am Rev Respir Dis 1987; 136:225–243.
14. Maesen FPV, Smeets JJ, Costongs MAL, Wald FDM, Cornelissen PJG. BA 679 BR, a new long-acting antimuscarinic bronchodilator: a pilot dose-escalation study. Eur Respir J 1993; 6:1031–1036.
15. Maesen FPV, Smeets JJ, Sledsens TJH, Wald FDM, Cornelissen PJG. Tiotropium bromide, a new long-acting antimuscarinic bronchodilator: a pharmacodynamic study in patients with chronic obstructive pulmonary disease (COPD). Eur Respir J 1995; 8:1506–1513.
16. Littner M, Auerbach D, Campbell S, Dunn L, Friedman M, Illowite J, Tashkin D, Taylor J, Menjoge S, Serby CW, Witek TJ Jr. The bronchodilator effects of tiotropium in stable COPD. Am J Respir Crit Care Med 1997; 155:A282.
17. Furguson GT, Cherniack RM. Management of chronic obstructive pulmonary disease. N Engl J Med 1993; 328:1017–1022.
18. Siafakas NM, Vermeire P, Pride NB, Paoletti P, Gibson J, Howard P, Yernault JC, Decramer M, Higgenbottom T, Postma DS, Rees J. Optimal assessment and management of chronic obstructive pulmonary disease (COPD). Eur Resp J 1995; 8:1398–1420.
19. Schuh S, Johnson DW, Callahan W, Canny G, Levison H. Efficacy of frequent nebulized ipratropium bromided added to frequent high-dose albuterol therapy in severe childhood asthma. J Pediatrics 1995; 126:639–645.
20. Garrett JE, Town L, Rodwell F, Kelly AM. Nebulized salmeterol with and without ipratropium bromide in the treatment of acute asthma. J Allergy Clin Immunol 1997; 100:165–170.
21. Ward MJ. The role of anticholinergic drugs in acute asthma. In: Cross NJ, ed. Anticholinergic Therapy in Obstructive Airways Disease. London: Franklin Scientific Publications, 1993:155–162.
22. Hayden FG, Diamond L, Wood PB, Forts D, Wecker MT. Effectiveness and safety of intranasal ipratropium bromide in common colds. Ann Intern Med 1996; 125:89–97.
23. Diamond L, Dockhorn RJ, Grossman J, Kisicki JC, Posner M, Zinny MA, Koker P, Korts D, Wecker MT. A dose-response study of the efficacy and safety of ipratropium bromide nasal spray in the treatment of common cold. J Allergy Clin Immunol 1995; 95:1139–1146.
24. Grossman J, Banov C, Boggs P, Bronsky EA, Dockhorn RJ, Druce H, Findlay SR, Georgitis JW, Hampel FC, Kaiser H, Ratner P, Tinkelman DG, Valentine MD, Roszko P, Zegarelli E, Wood C. Use of ipratropium bromide nasal spray in chronic treatment of nonallergenic perennial rhinitis, alone and in combination with other perennial rhinitis medications. J Allergy Clin Immunol 1995; 95: 1123–1127.
25. Meltzer E, Orgel A, Bronsky E, Findlay S, Georgitis J, Grossman J, Ratner P, Wood C. Ipratropium bromide aqueous nasal spray for patients with perennial allergic rhinitis: a study of its effect on their symptoms, quality of life, and nasal cytology. J Allergy Clin Immunol 1992; 90:242–245.

26. Anthonisen NR, Connett JE, Kiley JF, et al. Effects of smoking intervention and the use of an inhaled anticholinergic bronchodilator on the rate of decline of FEV_1. The Lung Health Study. JAMA 1994; 272:1497–1505.
27. Fryer AD, Wills-Karp M. Dysfunction of M_2-muscarinic receptors in pulmonary parasympathetic nerves after antigen challenge. J Appl Physiol 1991; 71:2255–2261.
28. Minette PAH, Lammers J, Dixon CMS, McCusker MT, Barnes PJ. A muscarinic agonist inhibits reflex bronchoconstriction in normal but not in asthmatic subjects. J Appl Physiol 1989; 67:2461–2465.
29. Ayala LE, Ahmed T. Is there a loss of a protective muscarinic receptor mechanism in asthma? Chest 1991; 96:1285–1291.
30. LeBlanc P, Bowie DM, Summers E, Jones NL, Killian KJ. Breathlessness and exercise in patients with cardiorespiratory disease. Am J Rev Respir Dis 1986; 133:21–25.
31. O'Donnell DE, Webb KA. Exertional breathlessness in patients with chronic airflow limitation. The role of lung hyperinflation. Am Rev Respir Dis 1993; 148:1351–1357.
32. Martin RJ, Smith P, Hudgel D, Lewis D, Pohl G, Souhrada JF. Ipratropium bromide (ATROVENT®) improves arterial oxygen saturation (SAO_2) in patients with COPD during sleep. Am J Resp Crit Care Med 1996; 153:A126.
33. Douglas NJ. Sleep. In: Calverly PMA, Pride NB, eds. Chronic Obstructive Pulmonary Disease. London: Chapman & Hall, 1995:293–308.
34. Chapman KR, Smith DL, Rebuck AS, Leenen FHH. Hemodynamic effects of inhaled ipratropium bromide, alone and combined with an inhaled $beta_2$-agonist. Am Rev Respir Dis 1985; 132:845–847.
35. Sackner MA, Friedman M, Silva G, Fernandez R. Pulmonary hemodynamic effects of aerosols of isoproterenol and ipratropium in normal subjects and patients with reversible airways obstruction. Am Rev Respir Dis 1977; 116:1013–1022.
36. Gross, NJ, Bankwala Z. Effects of an anticholinergic bronchodilator on arterial gases of hypoxemic patients with chronic obstructive pulmonary disease: comparison with a beta adrenergic agent. Am Rev Respir Dis 1987; 136:1091–1094.
37. Kalishker A, Nelson HE, Middleton E. Drug-induced changes of adenylate cyclase activity in cells from asthmatic and non asthmatic subjects. J Allergy Clin Immunol 1977; 60:259–265.
38. Barnes PJ. Circadian variation in airway function. Am J Med 1985; 79(suppl 6A):5–9.

Part Three

TOPICS OF SPECIAL INTEREST

9

Historical Aspects of Medicinal Uses of Antimuscarinics

KENNETH R. CHAPMAN

University of Toronto
Toronto, Ontario, Canada

I. Introduction

As millions of patients around the world inhale precisely metered quantities of antimuscarinic bronchodilator for relief of severe airflow obstruction, few would suspect that this modern and effective medication can trace its ancestry across centuries to the magical potions of Homeric legend. Crude botanical preparations of the deadly nightshade family (Solanaceae) have been used for millennia in cultures around the world. For most of their history, we have a record of these plant products being ingested deliberately or administered surreptitiously for their hallucinogenic and sometimes toxic properties.

Their more legitimate use as bronchodilators has a shorter documented history that still spans several centuries. Ayurvedic medical tradition of India recommended that the stems, leaves, and seeds of the plant be burned and the smoke inhaled for relief of respiratory symptoms. This practice was observed by British colonizers of the Indian subcontinent, who adopted it as the first inhaled bronchodilator therapy known to Western medicine. The inhalation of smoke from the burning Solanaceae became the mainstay of antiasthma therapy through the better part of the 19th century. When orthodox treatment in the 20th century turned its attention to the more rapidly acting adrenergic compounds and almost abandoned the anticholinergic agents, the folk practice of smoking anticholinergic asthma cigarettes survived in the patent medicine marketplace almost to the 21st century. Tracing the colorful history of these compounds, one is struck that our observant forebears had astutely outlined the principles of anticholinergic bronchodilator use well in advance of our modern pharmacologic science and clinical trial tools.

II. *Datura*

The *Datura* genus of the Solanaceae family is most closely associated with the medical history of antimuscarinics (1–3). Various species of the *Datura* genus grow worldwide and are usually considered weeds. In North America and Europe, the most common species of *Datura* is *Datura stramonium*, or Jimson weed. It was at one time called "the weed of civilization" for its propensity for rapid growth in farm yards, garbage heaps, and otherwise in close proximity to man. The plant has many other popular names including thornapple, devil's apple, mad apple of Peru, Stechapfel, pomme épineuse, and stinkweed (4). Although *D. stramonium* is the most often mentioned botanical source for the antimuscarinic bronchodilator therapy of the 19th century, other *Datura* species were widely available in other continents (5). *Datura ferox* was likely the original species smoked in India, where the British discovered the practice. In Africa and Asia, *Datura meteloides* grows widely and was likely known to the ancient Greeks for its possible medicinal and definite hallucinatory properties. The materia medica of China include the *Datura* species known as "man toe lo hua." In Japan, one member of the *Datura* genus is known as Yosku Chosenasagas. In Central and South America, *Datura inoxia*, *Datura candida*, *Datura sanguinea*, *Datura aurea*, and other *Datura* species figured prominently as hallucinogens used in religious ceremonies.

Datura stramonium can grow to considerable size, with 6 feet being common under ideal growing conditions. The plant has large, jagged, dark green leaves which have a heavy odor usually considered unpleasant. Its attractive trumpet-shaped flower is white or pale purple in color and is approximately 3 to 4 inches long. The trumpet-shaped Jimson weed flower opens in the evening; its shape accounts for other common names for the plant such as "angel trumpet" or "angel tulip." As the name "thornapple" suggests, the seedpod is a thorny capsule. This seedpod contains four cells, each filled with dark brown and wrinkled seeds approximately 2 to 3 mm long. When dry, the seed pod bursts to liberate hardy seeds that may survive for decades in the soil awaiting ideal conditions for germination. The entire plant from its root to its flower contains significant concentrations of belladonna alkaloids (hyoscyamine, hyoscine, atropine, and scopolamine).

III. Psychotropic Uses of Antimuscarinic Botanicals

Given their worldwide distribution, it is not surprising that these alkaloid-containing plants found their way into the medical folklore of many cultures. We do not know when they were first used in the treatment of airways diseases, but there is a long and colorful history of their use as intoxicants and hallucinogens.

The earliest literary reference to the use of *Datura* species for their psychotropic properties was plausibly a well-known episode in Homer's *Odyssey*. Although the Homeric legends are widely regarded as mythology, Graves has argued that they are poetic but historically accurate records of actual events (6). From this perspective Plaitakis and Duvoisin have argued that Odysseus' encounter with Circe is the first documented report of central nervous system poisoning by a plant, probably *Datura metaloides* (7). In Homer's recounting of the event, when Odysseus arrived at the island of Aeaea, Circe offered the crew food but "mixed in the food malignant drugs, so they might entirely forget their own fatherland . . . ." She then, as if by magic, changed the crew into pigs. The god Hermes warned Odysseus of these surreptitious poisons and offered Odysseus an antidote to the nymph's poison, the plant moly. Plaitakis and Duvoisin argue that the symptoms exhibited by Odysseus' crew resemble the delusional-hallucinatory state caused by the ingestion of belladonna alkaloids. Certainly, subsequent reports of poisoning (accidental or deliberate) by *Datura* plants describe a pronounced hallucinatory state sometimes lasting days followed by amnesia for the event (8). If Circe poisoned with *Datura* species, what was the antidote offered by the god Hermes? Moly may have been the plant "snowdrop" (*Galanthus nivalis*), which contains galanthamine, a centrally acting anticholinesterase.

Poisoning by *Datura* species has also figured prominently in other historical military campaigns. When Mark Anthony's legions retreated from Parthia in AD 38, they were said to have been poisoned by the surreptitious addition of *Datura* plants to their campfires. Inhaling the smoke of the campfires caused stupor and delirium. It is just as plausible that the Roman soldiers inadvertently added *Datura* species to their cook pots and that the ingestion of plant alkaloids caused stupor, coma, and death. Centuries later, in the New World, one such episode of inadvertent poisoning gave us the common name for *Datura stramonium*—Jimson weed. In 1676, British soldiers under the command of Captain John Smith were sent to Jamestown to prevent overthrow of the colonial government by the troops of Nathaniel Bacon (4). While foraging for food, Smith's troops inadvertently gathered up "Jamestown weed," or Jimson weed, to add to their food pots. Beverly's report of the incident describes clearly the hallucinogenic properties of ingesting belladonna alkaloids (1):

> The Jamestown Weed . . . being a early Plant, was gather'd very young for a boil'd salad, by some soldiers thither, to pacifie the troubles of Bacon; and some of them did eat plentifully of it, the effect of which was a very pleasant comedy; for they turned natural Fools upon it . . . . One would blow up a feather in the air; and another stark naked was sitting up in a Corner like a monkey grinning and making bows at them . . . . A thousand such simple tricks they play'd, and . . . returned to themselves again, not remembering anything that had passed . . . .

The 20th century saw military campaigns interrupted by *Datura* poisoning; during World War II, troops fighting in East Africa suffered wholesale poisoning by the same means as 17th-century British soldiers hoping to quell a colonial uprising in North America.

In the Americas, botanical sources of antimuscarinics were ingested deliberately for their hallucinogenic properties. For example, the Mohave's Pah-Utes drank extracts of *Datura stramonium* to produce intoxication as part of their religious ceremonies (3). Peruvian Indians ate or smoked the plant for religious reasons as well. As described by an early European explorer of Peru (9):

> The Indians believed that by drinking the tonga (*Datura*) they are brought into communication with their forefathers. I once had an opportunity of observing an Indian under the influence of this drink. Shortly after having swallowed the beverage he fell into a heavy stupor; he sat with his eyes vacantly fixed on the ground, his mouth convulsively closed and his nostrils dilated. In the course of about a quarter of an hour his eyes began to roll, foam issued from his half-open lips and his whole body was agitated by frightful convulsions. These violent symptoms having subsided, a profound sleep of several hours succeeded. In the evening . . . he alleged he had held communication with the spirits of his forefathers . . . .

Similar descriptions appear in the books of Carlos Castaneda in this century (10).

During the period of great geographical discoveries by Portuguese and Spanish navigators in the 15th and 16th centuries, explorations of the Americas and Asia taught Europeans the psychotropic uses of *Datura* species. At this time the hitherto unknown *Datura* species were first mentioned in the texts of Exotic Materia Medica. Some of the European authors not only observed the native use of these plants but grew them in their own botanical gardens. One such example is Garcia d'Orta (1501–1568) (11). d'Orta was the son of exiled Spanish Jews and studied arts and medicine at the Universities of Salamanca and Alcala de Henares. In 1554, he sailed to India as physician to the Portuguese Viceroy and participated in some of the Indian campaigns of conquest. He eventually settled to practice medicine in Goa, where he made many of his botanical observations. We remember d'Orta for his book *Colloquies on Simple Drugs . . . from India*, printed in Goa in 1563. d'Orta revealed information on the new Asian botanicals in the form of a dialogue between himself and a colleague, Ruano, who feigned ignorance of the new drugs. In one such dialogue, d'Orta describes a servant surreptitiously administering *Datura* to her mistress so that while her mistress was intoxicated she could rob the household of jewels and make good her escape. He reassures his colleague:

> There is no danger to the patient and all are cured within 24 hours. The people of this country do not consider this practice to be dangerous, nor do they think it is wrong except but when it is done with evil purposes. They do it to play a joke on someone, and I saw two men, the younger of them was 50 years old, to whom the sons of Nizamoxa gave it for fun, one was a hunter the other was a master maker of arrows and bows, and both were cured without any harm to their minds.

The psychotropic properties of stramonium were well known in European medical circles of the 18th and 19th centuries. Indeed, stramonium first entered the pharmacopoeia as a CNS drug used for the treatment of mania, depression, and even epilepsy (12). Trousseau and Pidoux describe with skepticism the use and presumed mechanism of action for stramonium in these various settings:

> Storck . . . 1762 . . . is considered the first that tried to utilize the active porperties of stramonium . . . . He treated five patients, two insane, one choreic, and two epileptic . . . . A considerable number of facts seem to confirm the value of stramonium in mania. Schneider . . . cured, slowly it is true, with tincture of stramonium, a lady of fifty years who suffered from demonomaniacal melancholy, and another woman who became mad after confinement . . . . Moreau . . . applies it chiefly to cases of monomania with hallucination, resting upon the fact that datura causes hallucinations, and that mania with hallucinations

ought to be cured by the drug in the same way that most irritants are used locally to cure irritation.

The consumption of anticholinergic botanicals has not always been benign. One must make note of their frequent use by assassins of the Middle Ages and later. Indeed, when Linne named the shrubs of the nightshade family, he used the name *Atropa belladonna*, invoking the name Atropose, the eldest of the three fates. According to mythology, Atropose cuts the thread of life.

The recreational use of anticholinergic botanicals has persisted to the modern era. As described below, patent medicine manufacturers offered atropine-containing or stramonium-containing asthma cigarettes for sale well into the 1960s and '70s. During the "psychedelic 60s," there were frequent reports in the medical literature of acute psychosis in teenagers and young adults seeking thrills by ingesting asthma cigarettes or smoking them to excess (5,8,13,14). There was widespread concern about the continued availability of these patent remedies, available over the counter and without a prescription.

IV. Anticholinergic Bronchodilators

The practice of inhaling anticholinergic bronchodilators (as smoke from burning plant leaves) may be 4 millennia old. Brewis describes papyrus records from the second millennium BC that document such practices (15). The papyrus records describe a problem of breathing compatible with asthma, and mention several remedies including henbane (*Hyoscyamus*). Inhalation therapy was also known to Greek physicians of Hippocrates' era. Indeed, Hippocrates believed that the afflicted body part should be treated directly with medication, and he therefore recommended vapor inhalation in the treatment of respiratory disease (16). The "metered dose inhaler" of the day was a lidded clay pot in which the stems and leaves of the plant were burned. A reed passed through a hole in the lid of the pot allowed the patient to inhale the medicinal vapors. Although we cannot document the use of *Datura* species specifically, it is possible that the plant found its way into these ancient Greek remedies. Our knowledge of non-Western folk remedies is limited, but Thai folk medicine of similar antiquity lists possible antimuscarinic botanicals among the favored remedies for asthma (17).

Gandevia has carefully documented the earliest clearly recorded use of botanical antimuscarinic treatment for airways disease (18). This practice was described in traditional Ayurvedic medicine of India. In the 17th-century Yogaratnakara, *Datura* is listed as a treatment for asthma although not without some questionable adjuvants: "One should powder together dry ginger, long pepper, black pepper, root of Datura plant and red arsenic, prepare paste out of it, turn in into a roll, dry it, and smoke it for three days.'' Mention has also been made of the possible use of *Datura* species by the Assyrians and even by native American Indians for the treatment of asthma.

The introduction of *Datura* remedies from Ayurvedic medicine into Western medicine may be credited to the astute powers of observation of Dr. James Anderson (1738–1809) (9). Anderson began his professional career in India, where he held the position of Physician-General of the East India Company at Madras. He rose from the lowly rank of assistant surgeon which he held in 1765 to membership of the medical board in 1800. In addition to pursuing his medical practice, he undertook projects in entomology, botany, and agriculture. A Renaissance man, he attempted to grow a variety of commercial plants such as sugar cane, coffee, American cotton, and European apples on the Indian subcontinent. He corresponded regularly with Sir Joseph Banks, president of the Royal Society, and described his scientific findings. He was also a pioneer in the medical field; in 1803, he was instrumental in introducing genuine cowpox into Hindustan with the goal of vaccinating against smallpox.

His experiments with *Datura ferox* may have been to treat his own respiratory disease. He had noted natives smoking dried and shredded roots of the plant for relief of breathing difficulties. After trying the material himself and feeling relief, he began to prescribe the botanical for his patients. He gave specimens of the plant to a General Gent who suffered from respiratory disease and apparently benefited from inhalation of *Datura* smoke. Upon Gent's return to Britain, he brought samples of the plant with him for his own use. In Edinburgh, Gent offered a sample of *Datura* to Dr. J. Sims. After undertaking a trial that confirmed his patients' enthusiastic report, Sims substituted the related local plant, *Datura stramonium*. This successful import from Indian medicine was described for the public in a letter to the editor of the *Monthly Magazine*. The letter was signed with the pseudonym Verox, but the writer was later identified as a London merchant, Mr. Sills. He describes ''great benefit'' from the use of this new medication. A more detailed medical description of *Datura*'s use appeared in the *Edinburgh Medical and Surgical Journal* authored by Dr. Sims. Early anecdotal reports of *Datura*'s efficacy were enthusiastic and uncritical, while orthodox medicine was more divided in its opinion. One enthusiast was Dr. William English, a surgeon who tried the remedy out of desperation for his own intractable asthma. He described the effect as ''wonderful—even to me almost incredible . . . the irritation and constant cough ceased . . . . I expectorated from the bronchia pieces of clear congealed phlegm, from half an inch to about an inch in length, and the thickness of a crow's quill . . . ." Some sober physicians felt this hyperbole to be incredible and said, "We should doubt its being related by a person educated in the medical profession" (20).

In mid-19th, century, Salter's *Treatise on Asthma* offered a balanced and thoughtful account of stramonium's uses, neglecting neither its dramatic benefits nor its significant hazard (21). Even while he quoted the enthusiastic praise of one patient ("in truth, the asthma is destroyed . . . . I would rather be without life than without stramonium . . ."), he reported that General Gent died while overusing *Datura stramonium*. He pointed out that in some instances "aggravation of the dyspnea" could result from its use, and he was mindful of potent central antimuscarinic effects. He listed among these "paralytic tremblings, epilepsy, headache, and apoplexy." Salter was greatly troubled by the sometimes contradictory results reported by the users of stramonium. Pondering this, he suggested that the potency of botanical preparations varied widely, depending on the native strength of the plant, its freshness, the method of its preparation, and its adulteration by adjuvants such as tobacco.

In a discussion reminiscent of our current debates concerning optimal inhalation devices, Salter also speculated that the specific method of inhalation might play a considerable role in the resulting therapeutic effect. Perhaps describing an early form of spacing chamber, he described one user of stramonium who "smoked . . . as you do tobacco then puffed the smoke into a tumbler, and then inhaled the cold smoke into his lungs." Salter's sober conclusions are noteworthy for their insight. He cautioned that stramonium was a quick-relief medication only and reported that "it has given only temporary relief—mitigated rather than cured the spasm." Cautioning those who would use it indiscriminately, he found:

> [Stramonium had] soon obtained as new remedies are apt to, the reputation of being specific and infallible;—everybody with any shortness of breathing was smoking stramonium . . . however . . . time has shaken it into its proper place, and assigned it its true worth;—that its original reputation greatly exaggerated its merit, but that it has undoubted though very unequal value, and will probably always maintain its place amongst the real remedies of asthma.

Salter had also noticed that diagnostic confusion might account for some of the suboptimal effects observed with stramonium. Much as we debate the differential diagnosis of asthma and COPD today, practitioners of the last century sought specific indication for anticholinergic bronchodilator therapy based upon specific categorizations in obstructive airways diseases. For example, in one prescient observation J. M. Fothergill, an Australian physiologist and physician, found that airways obstruction due to "emphysematous bronchitis'' responded particularly well to "fuming remedies" containing *Datura* (18,22). Waters, a contemporary of Fothergill, described the pathophysiology of emphysema accurately as a generalized loss of lung elastic recoil, and also found that particular benefit was likely to be had from the smoking of stramonium (18,23). (One must note with regret, however, that Waters also mentioned the potential benefits of smoking tobacco in the treatment of emphysema.)

By the late 19th century, stramonium was considered a mainstay of antiasthma therapy although various alternative therapies were also available. In an early edition of Osler's text, he noted:

> The sedative antispasmodics, such as belladonna, henbane, stramonium, and lobelia, may be given in solution or used in the form of cigarettes. Nearly all the popular remedies either in this form or in pastilles contain some plant of the order *solanaceae* [sic], with nitrate or chlorate of potash. Excellent cigarettes are now manufactured and asthmatics try various sorts, since one form benefits one patient, another form another patient (24).

Interest was not limited to English-speaking countries; various European nations used stramonium. As described by Trousseau and Pidoux, "*Datura stramonium* has not always succeeded in the hands of those who have tried it for . . . mania, epilepsy and chorea; but the incontestable value of the medicine in asthma . . . places it among those drugs on which therapeutics can best rely'' (12).

V. Antimuscarinic Therapy—Early Mechanistic Studies

Anticholinergic bronchodilators were inhaled centuries before it was understood how they worked. It's intriguing to speculate how the first user stumbled upon the useful medicinal properties of the smoke liberated by burning *Datura* leaves, but no explanation of antimuscarinic effect was possible before physicians had a sound understanding of pulmonary anatomy and physiology. In Antiquity and through the Middle Ages there were numerous fanciful accounts of how the breathing apparatus functioned and how it malfunctioned in cases of severe dyspnea (15,25). Our modern appreciation of how airway tone is controlled by the vagus nerve may be traced to the early 19th century. In 1808, Reisseissen described muscles encircling the bronchi and postulated that contraction of these muscles would produce airway narrowing and breathlessness. Until that time, it was more commonly believed that the airways expanded and contracted with each respiratory cycle. By 1830, Eberle had suggested that asthma was a consequence of vagal irritation with reflex contraction of bronchial musculature. Subsequently, Geiger and Hess isolated the active alkaloid daturine (atropine) from *Datura stramonium* (20).

Several medical investigators of the first half of the 19th century explored the role of the vagus nerve in asthma and other airway disorders. Among them, Charles J. B. Williams (1805–1889) offered useful data from a variety of animal studies (26). Williams studied medicine in Edinburgh and completed his M.D. thesis at the tender age of 19. He pursued further training with Laennec in Paris before becoming one of the eminent lung physicians of mid-19th-century London. Together with Sir Philip Rose, he founded the Brompton Hospital and he eventually served as president of both the Pathological Society and the New Sydenham Society. He also authored two major textbooks: *A Rational Exposition of the Physical Science of Diseases of the Chest*, and *Principles of Medicine*.

In various reports to the British Association for the Advancement of Science, Williams described the methods he used to study the contractility of bronchial smooth muscle. He performed experiments on dogs but also on rabbits, donkeys, and other livestock. The animal was usually killed by a blow to the head, but on numerous occasions the animal was sacrificed by the administration of morphine, stramonium, or belladonna. The lungs were excised along with a portion of the trachea. The trachea was then connected to a manometer filled with colored fluid. If Williams stimulated the trachea and bronchi using galvanic current, fluid rose in the manometer, allowing him to quantify the response to the applied stimulus. Although such stimulation usually produced a brisk rise in the manometer fluid, he observed that when dogs or rabbits had been killed with extracts of belladonna or stramonium, "Galvanism produced no effect for several minutes, and then a scarcely perceptible rise." This abolition of the usual response to electrical stimulation suggested a major role for cholinergic mechanisms in the maintenance of airway tone.

In subsequent studies, he generalized these observations to point out that esophageal and airway smooth muscle shared similar neural control mechanisms. In 1842, Longet offered dramatic evidence of the role of the vagus nerve by demonstrating bronchoconstriction following galvanic stimulation of the distal end of the cut vagus. Volkman replicated these experiments in large farm animals (and reported that the bronchoconstriction was sufficiently abrupt and large to blow out a candle). These experiments encouraged many to believe that asthma was the result of uncontrolled reflex bronchoconstriction, a neurogenic view of asthma that held sway for decades. In the middle to late 19th century, this view was supported by Salter and Osler among other prominent physicians. As described by Salter in his *Treatise on Asthma*: "If I were to express what appears to me the peculiar excellence of belladonna . . . in asthma I should say it consisted in its power of diminishing reflex irritability.''

VI. Efficacy of Asthma Cigarettes

Were the stramonium remedies of the last century and this century effective? This question was posed frequently by the middle of this century when accidental poisonings with asthma cigarettes seemed to outweigh their importance as legitimate asthma therapy. Asthma cigarettes remained popular patent medications despite little or no objective evidence of their benefit. Demonstration of bronchodilator benefit did not appear until the middle of the 20th century.

Harlow demonstrated that the cigarette was a most effective inhalation device (27). The average asthma cigarette liberated 0.5 mg of atropine in a fine aerosol of approximately 1-μm droplets. We understand today that the ideal droplet size for airway deposition is in the 2- to 5-μm range. The slightly smaller size of the asthma cigarette droplet suggests that there might have been considerable deposition in the lung periphery with consequent systemic absorption. By 1958, Ervenius and colleagues had pointed out the variable deposition of atropine in the lung and attributed this to the variable atropine content of available cigarettes as well as differences among individuals in inhalation technique (28). Even with cigarettes, "inhaler technique" was a significant factor influencing treatment outcome! These investigators recommended deep inhalation and breath holding, a technique described by Salter in his *Treatise* more than a century earlier.

Spirometry was finally used to quantify the benefit of stramonium cigarettes at approximately this time. Herxheimer described significant improvements in the vital capacity of asthmatics using asthma cigarettes (29). He carefully charted the pharmacodynamics of the atropine cigarette and reported that treatment effects were noticeable in as little as 3 to 5 min and were optimal at 30 min. The effect was transient, however, and disappeared in about 3 hours. As late as 1973, German investigators reported that asthma cigarettes available in that country could produce improvements in specific conductance comparable to those achieved by modern prescription medications (30). Very little work was done to investigate the systemic impact of antimuscarinic inhalation, but Elliot and Reed noted that the smoking of atropine-containing herbal cigarettes could produce a modest bradycardia similar to that produced by subtherapeutic doses of atropine (31). [The same effect has been described subsequently as a cardiovascular consequence of ipratropium inhalation from a metered-dose inhaler (32).]

By mid-20th century, few textbooks recommended antimuscarinic bronchodilator treatment although its role had been well documented in orthodox medical texts for over a century. Adrenergic therapy and xanthine therapy were considered the mainstays in the treatment of asthma and other obstructive airway diseases. However, adjunctive status was accorded the antimuscarinic bronchodilators. Typically administered in the form of atropine nebulization, investigators described possible additive benefits in severe cases of airways disease. For example, Hume and Rhys Jones noted that atropine inhalations could be used alone but worked more effectively in combination with isoprenaline (33). It remained for the introduction of quaternary anticholinergic derivatives in the latter 20th century for this adjunctive role to be reexamined in the setting of acute asthma and COPD (34,35).

VII. Modern Quaternary Antimuscarinics

The rediscovery of antimuscarinic bronchodilator therapy followed the introduction of safer, modern quaternary antimuscarinics. These compounds, poorly absorbed across biologic membranes, are relatively free from systemic absorption and are not associated with the side effects of General Gent's *Datura stramonium* or later patent remedies such as Asthmador cigarettes or Dr. Blosser's remedy.

The most widely studied of the quaternary anticholinergic bronchodilators, ipratropium, was first examined for its potential role in the treatment of asthma. It has become clear, however, that these agents have primarily an adjunctive role in the management of asthma whether chronic or acute. Their first-line bronchodilator status is reserved for older patients with chronic obstructive pulmonary disease. Astute clinicians and scientists of the last century suggested many of our current principles of optimal antimuscarinic bronchodilator therapy. Salter, for example, advised asthma patients to use stramonium before bedtime to reduce the risk of awakening with wheezing or cough in the early-morning hours (21). More recent studies with ipratropium have led to similar recommendations (36,37).

Similarly, Salter and his contemporaries did not overlook the psychogenic factors contributing to asthma. It has been suggested that modern quaternary antimuscarinics may be particularly effective for patients whose asthma is strongly influenced by psychogenic triggers (38). One principle of antimuscarinic therapy seems to have been overlooked by our forebears and may be considered a novel advance; the use of nasal ipratropium for vasomotor rhinitis has no 19th century corollary (39).

VIII. The Future of Antimuscarinic Bronchodilator Therapy

Our once-simple picture of cholinergic control mechanisms in the airway has been complicated by the discovery of muscarinic receptor subtypes (40). Muscarinic receptor structure has been clarified and muscarinic receptors have actually been cloned. Several different subtypes of muscarinic receptor have been identified, and this suggests the potential to develop selective and more potent antimuscarinic agents. M_3 receptors on bronchial smooth muscle contract when stimulated by acetylcholine. Hitherto unknown M_2 receptors on cholinergic nerve endings act as negative feedback receptors. That is, stimulation of M_2 receptors by acetylcholine blunts the release of neurotransmitters and diminishes cholinergic neural traffic. Available antimuscarinic agents such as ipratropium are nonselective in their action and block both M_3 and M_2 receptors. While blockade of the M_3 receptor subtype is clinically useful, blockade of the M_2 receptor subtype would diminish bronchodilator potency. Selective M_3 receptor blockers could prove more potent in the treatment of various airway diseases and could produce a renaissance of antimuscarinic bronchodilator therapy.

IX. Summary

Antimuscarinic agents have a long and colorful history spanning several continents and many cultures. Although there is a long and unsavory history of antimuscarinics as hallucinogens or poisons, their therapeutic history is almost as long. With the development of newer and perhaps more selective antimuscarinics it seems as likely today as in the last century that "[stramonium] will probably always maintain its place amongst the real remedies of asthma" (21).

References

1. Johnson CE. Mystical force of the nightshade. Int J Neuropsychiatry 1967; 3: 268–275.
2. Tramontana JA, Marderosian AH. Anti-asthmatic drugs as hallucinogens. Pennsylvania Med 1967; 70:58–60.
3. Hightower CE. Plants that kill and cure. Vet Hum Toxicol 1979; 21:360–362.
4. Thompson HS. Cornpicker's pupil: Jimson weed mydriasis. J Iowa Med Soc 1971; 61:475–478.
5. Chapman KR. History of anticholinergic treatment in airways disease. In: Gross

NJ, ed. Anticholinergic Therapy in Obstructive Airways Disease. London: Franklin Scientific Publications, 1993:9–17.
6. Graves R. The Greek Myths. Harmondsworth, U.K.: Penguin, 1960.
7. Plaitakis A, Duvoisin RC. Homer's moly identified as *Galanthus nivalis* L: physiologic antidote to stramonium poisoning. Clin Neuropharmacol 1983; 6:1–5.
8. Gowdy JM. Stramonium intoxication: review of symptomatology in 212 cases. JAMA 1972; 221:585–587.
9. Schultes RE. Peruvian and Chilean psychoactive plants mentioned in Ruiz's Relacion (1777–1788). J Psychoac Drugs 1983; 15:303–312.
10. Castaneda C. The Teachings of Don Juan: A Yaqui Way of Knowledge. Los Angeles: University of California Press, 1968.
11. Guerra F. Sex and drugs in the 16th century. Br J Addict 1974; 69:269–289.
12. Trousseau A, Pidoux H. Narcotics. In: Trousseau A, Pidoux H, eds. Treatise on Therapeutics. 9th ed. New York: William Wood & Company, 1880:217–295.
13. Ballantyne A, Lippiet P, Park J. Herbal cigarettes for kicks. BMJ 1976; 2:1539–1540.
14. Belton PA. Datura intoxication in West Cornwall. BMJ 1979; 1:585–586.
15. Brewis RAL. Classic Papers in Asthma. Vol. I. London: Science Press, 1992.
16. McFadden ER, Jr. Inhaled Aerosol Bronchodilators. Baltimore: Williams & Wilkins, 1986.
17. Panthong A, Kanjanapothi D, Taylor WC. Ethnobotanical review of medicinal plants Thai traditional books. Part 1. Plants with anti-inflammatory, antiasthmatic and antihypertensive properties. J Ethnopharmacol 1986; 18:213–228.
18. Gandevia B. Historical review of the use of parasympatholytic agents in the treatment of respiratory disorders. Postgrad Med J 1975; 51:13–20.
19. Cohen SG. James Anderson (1738–1809). Allergy Asthma Proc 1996; 17:165–167.
20. Hertz CW. Historical aspects of anticholinergic treatment of obstructive airways disease. Scand J Respir Dis 1979; suppl 103:105–109.
21. Salter HH. Treatment of the asthmatic paroxysm (continued)—treatment by stimulants. In: Anonymous. On Asthma: Its Pathology and Treatment. 1st ed. Philadelphia: Blanchard and Lea, 1864:134–144.
22. Fothergill JM. Chronic Bronchitis: Its Form and Treatment. London: Bailleire Tindall & Co., 1882.
23. Waters ATM. Researches on the Nature, Pathology and Treatment of Emphysema of the Lungs. London: Churchill, 1862.
24. Osler W. Diseases of respiratory system. In: Anonymous. The Principles and Practice of Medicine. 4th ed. New York: D. Appleton and Company, 1902:610–684.
25. Rosenblatt MB. History of bronchial asthma. In: Weiss EB, Segala C, eds. Bronchial Asthma: Mechanisms and Therapeutics. 1st ed. Boston: Little, Brown, 1976.
26. Lotvall J. Contractility of lungs and air-tubes: experiments performed in 1840 by Charles J.B. Williams. Eur Respir J 1994; 7:592–595.

27. Harlow ES. Some comments on temperature profiles throughout cigarettes, cigars and pipes. BMJ 1959; 2:167.
28. Ervenius O, Holmstedt B, Wallen O. Atropin-und Stramoniumzigaretten. Naunyn-Schmiedebergs Archiv fur Pharmakologie und Experimentelle Pathologie 1958; 234:343.
29. Herxheimer H. Atropine cigarettes in asthma and emphysema. BMJ 1959; 2: 167–171.
30. Trechsel K, Bachofen H, Scherrer M. Die bronchodilatorische Wirkung der Asthmazigarette. Schweiz Med Wochenschr 1973; 103:415.
31. Elliott HL, Reid JL. The clinical pharmacology of a herbal asthma cigarette. Br J Clin Pharmacol 1980; 10:487–490.
32. Chapman KR, Smith DL, Rebuck AS, Leenen FH. Hemodynamic effects of inhaled ipratropium bromide, alone and combined with an inhaled beta 2-agonist. Am Rev Respir Dis 1985; 132:845–847.
33. Hume KM, Rhys Jones E. The response to bronchodilators in intrinsic asthma. Q J Med 1961; 30:189.
34. Rebuck AS, Chapman KR, Abboud R, et al. Nebulized anticholinergic and sympathomimetic treatment of asthma and chronic obstructive airways disease in the emergency room. Am J Med 1987; 82:59–64.
35. Rebuck AS, Gent M, Chapman KR. Anticholinergic and sympathomimetic combination therapy of asthma. J. Allergy Clin Immunol 1983; 71:317–323.
36. Beakes DE. The use of anticholinergics in asthma. J. Asthma 1997; 34:357–368.
37. Coe CI, Barnes PJ. Reduction of nocturnal asthma by an inhaled anticholinergic drug. Chest 1986; 90:485–488.
38. Rebuck AS, Marcus HI. SCH 1000 in psychogenic asthma. Scand J Respir Dis 1979; suppl 103:186–191.
39. Grossman J, Banov C, Boggs P, et al. Use of ipratropium bromide nasal spray in chronic treatment of nonallergic perennial rhinitis, alone and in combination with other perennial rhinitis medications. J Allergy Clin Immunol 1995; 95 suppl: 1123–1127.
40. Gross NJ, Barnes PJ. A short tour around the muscarinic receptor. Am Rev Respir Dis 1988; 138:765–767.

10

Interaction of Virus with the Muscarinic Receptor

DAVID B. JACOBY

Bristol-Myers Squibb
Princeton, New Jersey

ALLISON D. FRYER

Johns Hopkins University
Baltimore, Maryland

I. Introduction

Viral infections of the airways commonly exacerbate asthma (1–5) and chronic bronchitis (6–11). In children at least 30% to 40% of asthma exacerbations are caused by viral infections (12–14). In a recent study in which children with asthma were followed for 2 years, viral infections were demonstrated in 80% of exacerbations (15) (Fig. 1). Improved, highly sensitive methods for detecting viral infections, coupled with collection of specimens at the earliest sign of an exacerbation, are likely to account for the high rate of association in this study.

In discussions of the role of viruses in acute asthma exacerbations, attention is often focused on virus-induced airway hyperresponsiveness. During viral infections, nonasthmatic patients become hyperresponsive both to nonspecific stimuli such as carbachol (1), histamine (16,17), citric acid (16), and exercise (18), and to inhalational challenge with specific antigen (17). The magnitude of these changes in nonspecific airway reactivity is small, and appears unlikely in itself to account for virus-induced asthma exacerbations. However, virus-induced changes in nonspecific airway responsiveness are vagally mediated (see below) and may reflect more important abnormalities in the vagal control of airway smooth muscle.

A variety of more specific, virus-induced changes in airway function appear more likely to contribute to the ability of these infections to exacerbate asthma. Both airway smooth muscle (19,20) and vascular responses (21) to tachykinins are potentiated by viral infections as viral infections decrease neutral endopeptidase, which normally degrades tachykinins. Similarly, virus-induced loss of airway histamine-N-methyltransferase may contribute to increased responsiveness to histamine (22). Viral infections may impair β-adrenoceptor function on airway smooth muscle, thereby reducing adrenergic relaxation (23,24). Nonadrenergic relaxation of the airways may also be reduced by viral infections (25).

A variety of pro-inflammatory effects of viruses may also be important. Leukocyte β-adrenoceptor function may be reduced during viral infections, impairing the ability of β-agonists to inhibit inflammatory cell function (26,27). Virus-infected airway epithelial cells release granulocyte-monocyte colony-stimulating factor, interleukin-6, interleukin-8, and RANTES (28–30), which can recruit and activate inflammatory cells. The inflammatory cells themselves can in turn respond to viruses by releasing many other important cytokines, including interferon-γ and MIP-1α (31). Epithelial cell production

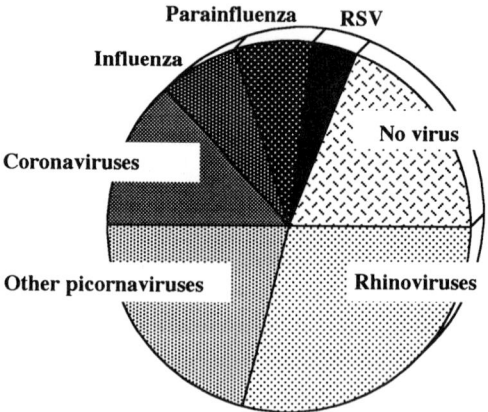

Figure 1 Viral infections accounted for 80% of asthma exacerbations in children ages 9 to 11 (15).

of interleukin-11 may increase nonspecific responsiveness and contribute to airway remodeling (32), while production of oxidant by epithelial cells and activated leukocytes may mediate tissue damage (33–35).

In terms of the functional changes leading to bronchoconstriction, a particularly potent effect of viral infections is to increase vagally mediated reflex bronchoconstriction. Changes in airway responsiveness after viral infection are often dependent on increased vagally mediated reflex bronchoconstriction. The increased airway response to exercise and to inhaled histamine can be reversed when the vagally mediated reflex component is eliminated (16,18). The response to histamine is also potentiated in virus-infected guinea pigs, and again an increased vagally mediated reflex is responsible as the hyperresponsiveness is eliminated by vagotomy (unpublished data). Changes in airway smooth muscle muscarinic receptors do not appear to be involved, as the airway tissues of animals with experimental viral infections are not hyperresponsive to acetylcholine in vitro (36). The mechanism appears to involve increased release of acetylcholine from vagal nerve endings (16,36).

II. Virus-Induced Parasympathetic Hyperresponsiveness

A. Naturally Occurring Viral Infections

There is substantial evidence of increased vagally mediated reflex bronchoconstriction in both experimental animals and humans with viral infections. Empey and colleagues (16) demonstrated that hyperresponsiveness to histamine in subjects with naturally occurring viral infections was vagally mediated, as the hyperresponsiveness was eliminated by pretreatment with atropine (Fig. 2). These investigators speculated that epithelial damage due to viral infection exposed irritant receptors, thus potentiating the afferent limb of the reflex arc. However, it was subsequently demonstrated (1) that parainfluenza virus infection in guinea pigs caused hyperresponsiveness to histamine that was vagally mediated, and (2) that the response to electrical stimulation of the vagus nerve was also increased in this model (36). Thus the efferent limb of the reflex arc is in fact increased by viral infection.

B. Muscarinic Receptor Subtypes in the Airways

The vagus nerve supplies the parasympathetic innervation of the lungs and airways. Acetylcholine is released from nerve endings onto excitatory muscarinic receptors on the airway smooth muscle. Stimulation of these receptors, which are of the M_3 subtype, causes smooth muscle contraction and bronchoconstriction. At the same time, released acetylcholine also feeds back onto

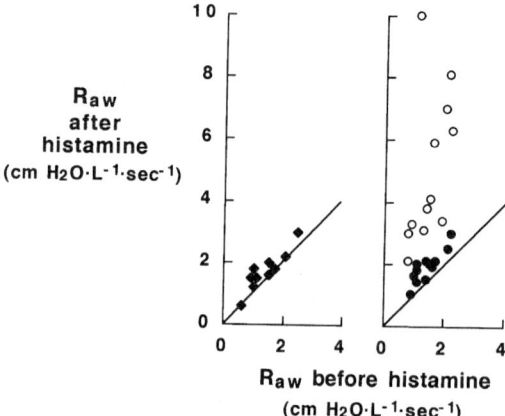

Figure 2 Airways resistance (R_{aw}) before and after a small dose of inhaled histamine (1.6%; 10 breaths). This dose did not increase R_{aw} in normal uninfected control subjects (left panel). In contrast, it did increase resistance in subjects with naturally occurring viral respiratory infections (right panel, open circles). Pretreating these patients with atropine (0.2%; 20 breaths) eliminated the hyperresponsiveness to histamine (right panel, closed circles). Thus the virus-induced hyperresponsiveness to histamine is due to a potentiated vagally mediated reflex bronchoconstriction (16).

inhibitory M_2 muscarinic receptors on the nerve ending itself (Fig. 3). This strong negative feedback limits further release of acetylcholine. Blocking the neuronal M_2 receptors with selective antagonists eliminates this negative feedback and potentiates vagally induced bronchoconstriction as much as 10-fold. Conversely, stimulating the inhibitory M_2 receptors with muscarinic agonists such as pilocarpine markedly decreases acetylcholine release and inhibits vagally mediated bronchoconstriction (37) (Fig. 4).

Inhibitory M_2 muscarinic receptors have been demonstrated in the airways of guinea pigs (37), rats (38), cats (39), dogs (40), and humans (41). Airway M_2 receptor function is impaired in some (42,43) but not all (44) patients with asthma.

Loss of neuronal M_2 receptor function in antigen-challenged guinea pigs increases vagally mediated bronchoconstriction (45). This increases the airway response to histamine only in animals with intact vagi. Preventing M_2 receptor dysfunction in these animals also prevents the development of airway hyperresponsiveness (46,47). Furthermore, acutely restoring M_2 receptor function

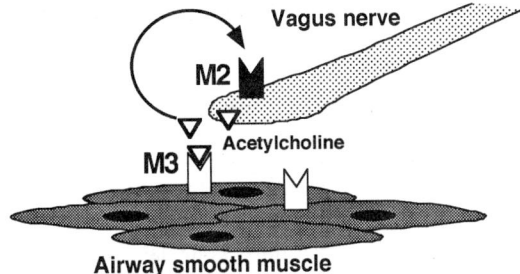

Figure 3 Acetylcholine is released from parasympathetic nerve endings in the airways and binds to M_3 receptors on the airway smooth muscle, stimulating smooth muscle contraction and bronchoconstriction. Acetylcholine also feeds back onto inhibitory M_2 receptors on the nerve ending itself, reducing the further release of acetylcholine.

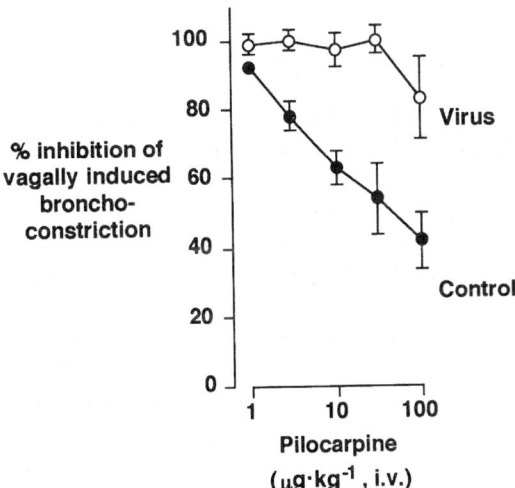

Figure 4 In uninfected guinea pigs (closed circles) pilocarpine stimulates inhibitory M_2 receptors on the parasympathetic nerve endings, reducing acetylcholine release and inhibiting the bronchoconstriction response to electrical stimulation of the vagus. In contrast, pilocarpine has little effect on the response to vagal stimulation in guinea pigs that are infected with parainfluenza virus (open circles), demonstrating loss of function of the M_2 receptors on the nerves (50).

in antigen-challenged animals immediately reverses airway hyperresponsiveness (48,49).

C. M_2 Receptor Dysfunction During Viral Infections

Because loss of M_2 receptor function increases the release of acetylcholine, thereby potentiating vagally mediated reflex bronchoconstriction by enhancing the efferent limb of this reflex arc, we investigated M_2 receptor function in parainfluenza virus-infected guinea pigs. Four days after infection, we tested the ability of the muscarinic agonist pilocarpine to inhibit the in vivo bronchoconstriction response to electrical stimulation of the vagus nerves. In uninfected animals, pilocarpine inhibited vagally mediated bronchoconstriction in dose-dependent fashion. In contrast, this effect of pilocarpine was largely lost in virus-infected guinea pigs (Fig. 4) (50). Thus viral infection causes M_2 receptor dysfunction, increasing the release of acetylcholine and potentiating vagally mediated bronchoconstriction. Similar dysfunction of neuronal inhibitory M_2 muscarinic receptors has been demonstrated after parainfluenza infections in rats (51).

D. Glycosylation of the M_2 Receptor

The M_2 receptor is N-glycosylated at three asparagine residues (Asn^2, Asn^3, and Asn^6) in the extracellular portion of the receptor. Carbohydrates make up 26.5% of the molecular weight of the receptor (52). Gies and Landry (53) showed that treatment of M_2 receptors with the enzyme neuraminidase, which cleaves the sialic acid residues from the receptor, decreases the affinity of muscarinic agonists for the M_2 receptor but not for other muscarinic receptor subtypes.

Neuraminidase is contained in the coat of both influenza and parainfluenza viruses (54) and is expressed in large quantities in infected tissues (55). We demonstrated that incubation of M_2 muscarinic receptors in vitro with parainfluenza virus did not affect the number of receptors, but did decrease the agonist affinity by an order of magnitude (56). This effect was mimicked by an equivalent concentration of *Clostridium perfringens* neuraminidase, and the effect of virus was blocked by 2,3-dehydro-2-deoxy-N-acetyl-neuraminic acid (DDN), an inhibitor of neuraminidase.

We performed similar studies using a membrane preparation of guinea pig lung. In untreated lung, carbachol displaced ligand from two sites (Hill coefficient = 0.53)—a high-affinity site with K_D = 0.21μM (31% of sites), and a low-affinity site with K_D = 15 μM (69% of sites). After exposure to neuraminidase, the agonist affinity of the high-affinity site was decreased by an order of magnitude, so that it became indistinguishable from the low-affinity site. The low-affinity site was unaffected. When virus was substituted for neuraminidase, a similar shift in the agonist affinity of the high-affinity site resulted. The neuraminidase inhibitor DDN prevented this shift. The contribution of M_2 and M_3 receptors to the high- and low-affinity binding sites is not known, but it is possible to state on the basis of these experiments that neuraminidase, which affects M_2 receptor agonist affinity, decreased the agonist affinity of a subpopulation of lung muscarinic receptors.

E. Inflammatory Responses to Viral Infections

To determine the role of inflammation in virus-induced M_2 receptor dysfunction, we pretreated guinea pigs with cyclophosphamide (30 mg · kg^{-1}) daily for 7 days, after which we infected them with parainfluenza virus. Four days later we tested their response to vagal stimulation and to pilocarpine and gallamine. Of 10 guinea pigs studied, cyclophosphamide protected M_2 receptor function in four animals despite viral infection. The remaining six lost M_2 receptor function despite being depleted of leukocytes as determined by both peripheral blood and lung lavage cell counts.

Because virus may replicate to higher levels in the lungs of leukocyte-depleted animals (57,58), we determined the viral content of the lungs in this experiment. Guinea pigs that lost M_2 receptor function despite leukocyte depletion had significantly greater lung viral content than those that retained normal M_2 receptor function. The viral titers in both groups overlapped those of non-leukocyte-depleted animals (59).

Thus viral infection causes M_2 receptor dysfunction via multiple mechanisms. In animals with mild infections, M_2 receptor function is the result of the inflammatory response to the infection. In more severe infections, the virus is able to cause loss of M_2 receptor function in the absence of an inflammatory response.

F. Role of Tachykinins in Virus-Induced M_2 Receptor Dysfunction

Viral infections potentiate many effects of tachykinins by decreasing the activity of airway neutral endopeptidase, an enzyme that breaks down tachykinins (19). Because tachykinins recruit and activate inflammatory cells (60,61), we tested the effects of neurokinin receptor antagonists on virus-induced inflammation and M_2 receptor dysfunction. Blocking NK1 receptors did not affect the inflammatory response to subsequent parainfluenza infection, but did prevent virus-induced M_2 receptor dysfunction (62). The mechanism of this effect is not known, but may be related to prevention of leukocyte activation.

G. M₂ Receptor Gene Expression and Function in Cultured Airway Parasympathetic Neurons

In order to further explore the mechanisms of virus-induced M_2 receptor dysfunction, we developed a method for growing airway parasympathetic neurons in culture. These cells retain a nerve cell-like morphology, synthesize acetylcholine and release it in response to electrical stimulation, and express a functional M_2 muscarinic receptor (63). Thus exposing these cells to the muscarinic agonist methacholine suppresses the release of acetylcholine, while treating the cells with atropine blocks the M_2 receptor and increases acetylcholine release.

Exposing these cells to parainfluenza virus results in infection of the neurons as demonstrated by production of progeny virus and expression of viral antigen on the cell membrane (64). In both virus-infected cells and neurons exposed to interferon-γ (which is produced by lymphocytes in response to viral infections), release of acetylcholine in response to electrical stimulation was potentiated. Furthermore, methacholine was no longer able to suppress the release of acetylcholine, while atropine no longer potentiated it (Fig. 5). Thus the M_2 receptor on these cells was no longer functional.

We used a competitive reverse transcription polymerase chain reaction assay to quantify expression of the gene for the M_2 muscarinic receptor in these neurons. Loss of receptor function was accompanied by a 10-fold or greater decrease in receptor gene expression in both virus-infected and interferon-treated cells. It may also be significant that dexamethasone increases M_2 receptor gene expression and blocks the loss of M_2 receptor gene expression in interferon-γ-treated cells (65).

H. Interactions Between Atopy and Viral Infections: The Role of the Eosinophil

Animals that are sensitized to an antigen and then challenged with that antigen via inhalation also lose neuronal M_2 receptor function. In this case, it is clearly the eosinophil that is responsible for M_2 receptor dysfunction. In these animals, eosinophils are recruited selectively into the airway nerve bundles, parasympathetic ganglia, and nerve fibers (66). A similar association of eosinophils with the nerves is found in the airways of patients that have died with acute asthma (66). In antigen-challenged guinea pigs, blocking the eosinophil influx into the airway by depleting eosinophils by treating the animals with antibodies to either interleukin-5 (67) or the eosinophil adhesion molecule VLA-4 (46) prevents M_2 receptor dysfunction and hyperresponsiveness in these animals (46,68).

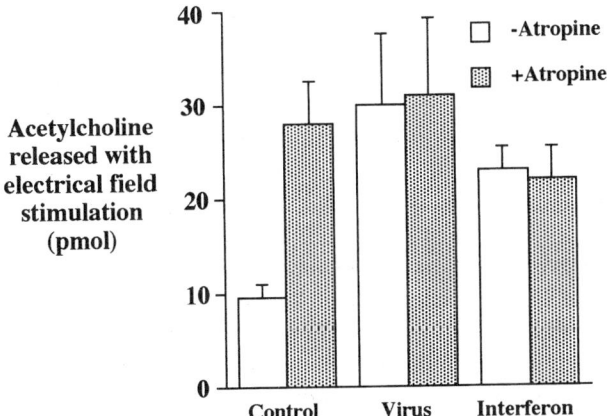

Figure 5 In cultured airway parasympathetic neurons, acetylcholine is released by electrical stimulation. When M_2 receptors on the neurons are blocked with atropine, the negative feedback normally provided by these receptors is eliminated, and acetylcholine release is increased. In cells that are infected with parainfluenza virus or exposed to interferon-γ (300 U/mL), M_2 receptor function is lost and acetylcholine release is increased. In these cells, atropine does not cause further increase in acetylcholine release, as the M_2 receptor is already nonfunctional (64).

It is specifically the eosinophil major basic protein that, by acting as an M_2 muscarinic receptor antagonist (69), causes the M_2 receptor dysfunction and subsequent hyperresponsiveness. Pretreating animals with an antibody to major basic protein prevents antigen-induced M_2 receptor dysfunction without inhibiting recruitment of eosinophils to the nerves (47). Furthermore, any of several polyanionic substances that bind major basic protein (including heparin, partially desulfated heparin, and poly-L-glutamic acid) can acutely reverse M_2 receptor dysfunction and hyperresponsiveness in antigen-challenged animals (48,49).

In contrast, viral infections do not generally cause airway eosinophilia, and antibody to interleukin-5 does not prevent virus-induced M_2 receptor dysfunction (unpublished observation). Furthermore, heparin, which reverse both hyperresponsiveness and M_2 receptor dysfunction after antigen challenge, does not reverse virus-induced M_2 receptor dysfunction (59). Thus neither eosinophils nor major basic protein is responsible for M_2 receptor dysfunction in virus-infected animals.

Airway viral infections have traditionally been thought to cause a neutrophil influx into the airways followed by a mononuclear cell influx (70) and to elicit a predominantly CD8+ T-lymphocyte response (71), yielding interferon-γ as an important anti-viral cytokine (72). A CD4+ T-lymphocyte response may also contribute to viral clearance, and here again it is production of interferon-γ by TH1 cells that appears to be beneficial (73).

Under normal circumstances, eosinophils are not prominent in the response to most airway viruses. It has become apparent, however, that under specific conditions, viral infections are capable of producing a varied inflammatory response, including airway eosinophilia and production of interleukin-5 by both CD8+ and CD4+ T-lymphocytes. It has been shown that while under normal circumstances CD8+ T-lymphocytes produce interferon-γ in response to viral infections, in an allergic milieu these CD8+ cells respond to viral infections by producing interleukin-5 (74,75). Studies by Coyle et al. (75) used a transgenic mouse model in which the CD8+ T-lymphocytes expressed the receptor for a particular viral glycoprotein. When these mice inhaled this glycoprotein, their lung lavage demonstrated production of interferon-γ and an influx of neutrophils and mononuclear cells. However, if the mice were first sensitized to an irrelevant antigen (ovalbumin, given intraperitoneally), the response to inhaled viral glycoprotein was production of interleukin-5 and an influx of eosinophils. These investigators demonstrated that exposure of the transgenic CD8+ T-lymphocytes to interleukin-4 changed their in vitro response to viral glycoprotein from interferon-γ to interleukin-5. Thus it was postulated that in an ''atopic'' animal (i.e., one that had been sensitized to ovalbumin), production of interleukin-4 conditioned the CD8+ T-lymphocytes so that their response to viral antigen was to produce interleukin-5 and to promote pulmonary eosinophilia.

It has also been demonstrated that CD4+ T-lymphocytes, while generally responding to viral infections by differentiating toward a TH1 phenotype, can also respond by becoming TH2 cells (73). This response was demonstrated in influenza infections of mice, in which a TH2 response caused pulmonary eosinophilia, increased lung damage, and delayed viral clearance.

Eosinophils and their proteins have been recovered from both humans and mice with viral infections (76–78). In allergic humans, experimental rhinovirus infections increase the recruitment of eosinophils to the airways after antigen challenge (79). In view of the association of eosinophils with asthma and asthma exacerbations (80) and the strong association of asthma exacerbations with viral infections, we postulated that this eosinophil influx may be an important mechanism of virus-induced asthma and loss of M_2 receptor function.

To explore the possibility that the inflammatory response to viral infection and the mechanisms of M_2 receptor dysfunction might be different in an atopic (i.e., antigen-sensitized) animal, we sensitized guinea pigs to ovalbumin via intraperitoneal injection (81). Two weeks later we infected them with parainfluenza virus given intranasally. No ovalbumin was delivered into the airways. These animals developed M_2 receptor dysfunction, but, in contrast to nonsensitized animals, in which the predominant inflammatory cell in the airway was the neutrophil, the sensitized animals developed airway eosinophilia in response to viral infection. Furthermore, while heparin did not restore M receptor function in nonsensitized, virus-infected animals, heparin did restore M_2 receptor function in sensitized virus-infected animals. Thus the airway eosinophils and major basic protein were responsible for M_2 receptor dysfunction in antigen-sensitized, virus-infected animals. This may be relevant to the airway hyperresponsiveness, airway eosinophilia, and exacerbations of asthma experienced by atopic asthmatics during viral infections.

I. Postrecovery Changes in M_2 Receptor Function

During recovery from viral infections, M_2 receptor function returns to normal after 2 to 4 weeks (82,83). However, while M_2 receptor function in pathogen-free guinea pigs is not dependent on production of cyclo-oxygenase products, after recovery from viral infections M_2 receptor function can be completely blocked by indomethacin (83). The mechanisms of this change in receptor coupling, and its possible significance in aspirin-sensitive asthma, are unknown.

III. Conclusion

Viral infections are a major cause of asthma attacks. A particularly important cause of bronchoconstriction appears to be increased vagally mediated bronchoconstriction. Loss of inhibitory M_2 muscarinic receptor function on airway parasympathetic nerve endings increases acetylcholine release, potentiating reflex bronchoconstriction and mediating hyperresponsiveness. A variety of effects of the virus itself and of the inflammatory response to the infections contribute to M_2 receptor dysfunction, and may lead both to loss of function and to loss of expression of the receptor. In addition, the allergic status of the host may alter both the inflammatory response to the virus and the mechanism of M_2 receptor dysfunction, with an allergic host experiencing an influx of eosinophils, which then release major basic protein which acts as an M_2 receptor antagonist. Binding the major basic protein using polyanionic substances restores M_2 receptor function and eliminates vagally mediated hyperresponsiveness, suggesting that this may be a therapeutic opportunity.

References

1. Little JW, Hall WJ, Douglas RG, Mudholkar GS, Speers DM, Patel K. Airway hyperreactivity and peripheral airay dysfunction in influenza A infection. Am Rev Respir Dis 1978; 118:295–303.
2. Frick OL, German DF, Mills J. Development of allergy in children. I. Association with virus infections. J Allergy Clin Immunol 1979; 63:228–241.
3. Henderson FW, Clyde WA, Collier AM, et al. The etiologic and epidemiologic spectrum of bronchiolitis in pediatric practice. J Pediatr 1979; 95:183–190.
4. Welliver RC. Upper respiratory infections in asthma. J Allergy Clin Immunol 1983; 72:341–346.
5. Frick WE, Busse WW. Respiratory infections: their role in airway responsiveness and pathogenesis of asthma. Clin Chest Med 1988; 9:539–549.
6. Carilli AD, Gohd RS, Gordon W. A virological study of chronic bronchitis. N Engl J Med 1964; 270:123–127.
7. Eadie MB, Stott EJ, Grist NR. Virological studies in chronic bronchitis. Br Med J 1966; 2:671–673.
8. Stenhouse AC. Rhinovirus infection in acute exacerbations of chronic bronchitis. Br Med J 1967; 3:461–463.
9. Stenhouse AC. Viral antibody levels and clinical status in acute exacerbations of chronic bronchitis: a controlled prospective study. Br Med J 1968; 3:287–290.
10. Lamy ME, Pouthier-Simon F, Debaker-Williame E. Respiratory viral infections in hospital patients with chronic bronchitis. Chest 1973; 63:336–341.
11. Gump DW, Phillips CA, Forsyth BR, McIntosh K, Lamborn KR, Stouch WH. Role of infection in chronic bronchitis. Am Rev Respir Dis 1976; 113:465–474.
12. McIntosh K, Ellis EF, Hoffman LS, Lybass TG, Eller JJ, Fulginiti VA. The association of viral and bacterial respiratory infections with exacerbations of wheezing in young asthmatic children. J Pediatr 1973; 82:578–590.
13. Minor TE, Dick EC, DeMeo AN, Ouellette JJ, Cohen M, Reed CE. Viruses as precipitants of asthmatic attacks in children. JAMA 1974; 227:292–298.
14. Minor TE, Dick EC, Baker JW, Ouellette JJ, Cohen M, Reed CE. Rhinovirus and influenza type A infections as precipitants of asthma. Am Rev Respir Dis 1976; 113:149–153.
15. Johnston SL, Pattemore PK, Sanderson G, et al. Community study of role of viral infections in exacerbations of asthma in 9–11 year old children. Br Med J 1995; 310(6989):1225–1229.
16. Empey DW, Laitinen LA, Jacobs L, Gold WM, Nadel JA. Mechanisms of bronchial hyperreactivity in normal subjects following upper respiratory tract infection. Am Rev Respir Dis 1976; 113:523–527.
17. Lemanske RF, Dick EC, Swensen CA, Vrtis RF, Busse WW. Rhinovirus upper respiratory infection increases airway hyperreactivity and late asthmatic reactions. J Clin Invest 1989; 83:1–10.

18. Aquilina AT, Hall WJ, Douglas RG, Utell MJ. Airway reactivity in subjects with viral upper respiratory tract infections: the effects of exercise and cold air. Am Rev Respir Dis 1980; 122:3–10.
19. Jacoby DB, Tamaoki J, Borson DB, Nadel JA. Influenza infection causes airway hyperresponsiveness by decreasing enkephalinase. J Appl Physiol 1988; 64(6): 2653–2658.
20. Dusser DJ, Jacoby DB, Djokic TD, Rubenstein I, Borson DB, Nadel JA. Virus induces airway hyperresonsiveness to tachykinins: role of neutral endopeptidase. J Appl Physiol 1989; 67:1504–1511.
21. Piedimonte G, Umeno E, McDonald DM, Nadel JA. Sendai virus infection potentiates neurogenic inflammation in the rat-trachea. Am Rev Respir Dis 1989; 139:A230.
22. Nakazawa H, Sekizawa K, Morikawa M, et al. Viral respiratory infection causes airway hyperresponsiveness and decreases histamine N-methyltransferase activity in guinea pigs. Am J Respir Crit Care Med 1994; 149(5):1180–1185.
23. Scarpace PJ, Bender BS. Viral pneumonia attenuates adenylate cyclase but not beta-adrenergic receptors in murine lung. Am Rev Respir Dis 1989; 140:1602–1606.
24. Henry PJ, Rigby PJ, Mackenzie JS, Goldie RG. Effect of respiratory tract viral infection on murine airway B-adrenoceptor function, distribution, and density. Br J Pharmacol 1991; 104:914–921.
25. Colasurdo GN, Hemming VG, Prince GA, Loader JE, Graves JP, Larsen GL. Human respiratory syncytial virus affects nonadrenergic noncholinergic inhibition in cotton rat airways. Am J Physiol 1995; 268(6 Pt 1):L1006–L1011.
26. Busse WW, Anderson CL, Dick EC, Warshauer D. Reduced granulocyte response to isoproterenol, histamine, and prostaglandin E1 after in vitro incubation with rhinovirus 16. Am Rev Respir Dis 1980; 122:641–646.
27. Buckner CK, Clayton DE, Ain-Shoka AA, Busse WW, Dick EC, Shult P. Parainfluenza 3 infection blocks the ability of a beta adrenergic receptor to inhibit antigen-induced contraction of guinea pig isolated airway smooth muscle. J Clin Invest 1981; 67:376–384.
28. Choi AMK, Jacoby DB. Influenza virus A infection induces interleukin-8 gene expression in human airway epithelial cells. FEBS Lett 1992; 309:327–329.
29. Subauste MC, Jacoby DB, Proud D. Infection of a human respiratory epithelial cell line with rhinovirus. Induction of cytokine release and modulation of susceptibility to infection by cytokine exposure. J Clin Invest 1995; 96:549–557.
30. Becker S, Reed W, Henderson FW, Noah TL. RSV infection of human airway epithelial cells causes production of the beta-chemokine RANTES. Am J Physiol 1997; 272(3 Pt 1):L512–L520.
31. Cook DN, Beck MA, Coffman TM, et al. Requirement of MIP-1 alpha for an inflammatory response to viral infection. Science 1995; 269(5230):1583–1585.
32. Elias JA, Zheng T, Einarsson O, et al. Epithelial interleukin-11. Regulation by cytokines, respiratory syncytial virus, and retinoic acid. J Biol Chem 1994; 269(35):22261–22268.

33. Oda T, Akaike T, Hamamoto T, Suzuki F, Hirano T, Maeda H. Oxygen radicals in influenza-induced pathogenesis and treatment with pyran polymer-conjugated SOD. Science 1989; 244:974–976.
34. Akaike T, Ando M, Oda T, et al. Dependence on O^-_2 generation by xanthine oxidase of pathogenesis of influenza virus infection in mice. J Clin Invest 1990; 85:739–745.
35. Knobil K, Choi AMK, Weigand GW, Jacoby DB. Role of oxidants in influenza virus-induced gene expression. Am J Physiol Lung Cell Mol Physiol 1998; 274: L134–L142.
36. Buckner CK, Songsiridej V, Dick EC, Busse WW. In vivo and in vitro studies of the use of the guinea pig as a model for virus-provoked airway hyperreactivity. Am Rev Respir Dis 1985; 132:305–310.
37. Fryer AD, Maclagan J. Muscarinic inhibitory receptors in pulmonary parasympathetic nerves in the guinea-pig. Br J Pharmacol 1984; 83:973–978.
38. Aas P, Maclagan J. Evidence for prejunctional M_2 muscarinic receptors in pulmonary cholinergic nerves of the rat. Br J Pharmacol 1990; 101:73–76.
39. Blaber LC, Fryer AD, Maclagan J. Neuronal muscarinic receptors attenuate vagally-induced contraction of feline bronchial smooth muscle. Br J Pharmacol 1985; 86:723–728.
40. Ito Y, Yoshitomi T. Autoregulation of acetylcholine release from vagus nerves terminals through activation of muscarinic receptors in the dog trachea. Br J Pharmacol 1988; 93:636–646.
41. Minette P, Barnes PJ. Prejunctional inhibitory muscarinic receptors on cholinergic nerves in human and guinea-pig airways. J Appl Physiol 1988; 64:2532–2537.
42. Minette PJ, Lammers JWJ, Dixon CMS, McCusker MT, Barnes PJ. A muscarinic agonist inhibits reflex bronchoconstriction in normal but not asthmatic subjects. J Appl Physiol 1989; 67:2461–2465.
43. Ayala LE, Ahmed T. Is there loss of a protective muscarinic receptor in asthma? Chest 1989; 96:1285–1291.
44. Okayama M, Shen T, Midorikawa J, et al. Effect of pilocarpine on propranolol-induced bronchoconstriction in asthma. Am J Respir Crit Care Med 1994; 149(1): 76–80.
45. Fryer AD, Wills-Karp M. Dysfunction of M_2 muscarinic receptors in pulmonary parasympathetic nerves after antigen challenge in guinea-pigs. J Appl Physiol 1991; 71:2255–2261.
46. Fryer AD, Costello RW, Yost BL, et al. Antibody to VLA-4, but not to L-selectin, protects neuronal M_2 muscarinic receptors in antigen-challenged guinea pig airways. J Clin Invest 1997; 99(8):2036–2044.
47. Evans CM, Jacoby DB, Gleich GJ, Fryer AD, Costello RW. Antibody to eosinophil major basic protein protects M_2 receptor function of antigen challenged guinea pigs in vivo. J Clin Invest 1997; 100:2254–2262.
48. Fryer AD, Jacoby DB. Function of pulmonary M_2 muscarinic receptors in antigen challenged guinea-pigs is restored by heparin and poly-l-glutamate. J Clin Invest 1992; 90:2292–2298.

49. Fryer A, Huang YC, Rao G, et al. Selective O-desulfation produces nonanticoagulant heparin that retains pharmacological activity in the lung. J Pharmacol Exp Ther 1997; 282(1):208–219.
50. Fryer AD, Jacoby DB. Parainfluenza virus infection damages inhibitory M_2 muscarinic receptors on pulmonary parasympathetic nerves in the guinea-pig. Br J Pharmacol 1991; 102:267–271.
51. Sorkness R, Clough JJ, Castleman WL, Lemanske RF. Virus-induced airway obstruction and parasympathetic hyperresponsiveness in adult rats. Am J Respir Crit Care Med 1994; 150(1):28–34.
52. Peterson GL, Rosenbaum LC, Broderick DJ, Schimerlik MI. Physical properties of the purified cardiac muscarinic acetylcholine receptor. Biochemistry 1986; 25: 3189–3202.
53. Gies J-P, Landry Y. Sialic acid is selectively involved in the interaction of agonists with M_2 muscarinic acetylcholine receptors. Biochem Biophys Res Commun 1988; 150:673–680.
54. Scheid A, Caliguiri LA, Compans RW, Choppin PW. Isolation of paramyxovirus glycoproteins. Association of both hemagglutinating and neuraminidase activities with the larger SV5 glycoprotein. Virology 1972; 50:640–652.
55. Boulan ER, Pendergast M. Polarized distribution of viral envelope proteins in the plasma membrane of infected epithelial cells. Cell 1980; 20:45–54.
56. Fryer AD, El-Fakahany EE, Jacoby DB. Parainfluenza virus type 1 reduces the affinity of agonists for muscarinic receptors in guinea-pig heart and lung. Eur J Pharmacol 1990; 181:51–58.
57. Singer SH, Ford M, Kirschstein RL. Respiratory diseases in cyclophosphamide-treated mice. II. Decreased virulence of PR8 influenza virus. Infect Immun 1972; 5:957–960.
58. Hurd J, Heath RB. Effect of cyclophosphamide on infections in mice caused by virulent and avirulent strains of influenza virus. Infect Immun 1975; 11:886–889.
59. Fryer AD, Yarkony KA, Jacoby DB. The effect of leukocyte depletion on pulmonary M_2 muscarinic receptor function in parainfluenza virus-infected guinea-pigs. Br J Pharmacol 1994; 112:588–594.
60. Bar-Shavit Z, Goldman R, Stubinsky Y, et al. Enhancement of phagocytosis-A newly found activity of substance P residing in its N-terminal tetrapeptide sequence. Biochem Biophys Res Commun 1980; 4:1445–1451.
61. Marasco WA, Showell HJ, Becker EL. Substance P binds to the formylpeptide chemotaxis receptor on the rabbit neutrophil. Biochem Biophys Res Commun 1981; 99:1065–1072.
62. Elwood T, Jacoby DB, Fryer AD. Virus-induced airway inflammation and loss of inhibitory M_2 muscarinic receptor functions is prevented by pretreatment with a neurokinin-1 receptor anatagonist. Am J Respir Crit Care Med 1998; 157:A210.
63. Fryer AD, Elbon CL, Kim AL, Xiao H-Q, Levey AI, Jacoby DB. Cultures of airway parasympathetic nerves express functional M_2 muscarinic receptors. Am J Respir Cell Mol Biol 1996; 15:716–725.

64. Jacoby DB, Xiao HQ, Lee NH, Chan-Li Y, Fryer AD. Virus- and interferon-induced loss of inhibitory M_2 muscarinic receptor function and gene expression in cultured airway parasympathetic neurons. J Clin Invest 1998; 102:242–248.
65. Jacoby DB, Chani-Li Y, Xiao HQ, Fryer AD. Dexamethasone increases M_2 muscarinic receptor expression and decreases acetylcholine release in cultured airway parasympathetic neurons. Am J Respir Crit Care Med 1998; 157:A715.
66. Costello RW, Schofield BH, Kephart GM, Gleich GJ, Jacoby DB, Fryer AD. Localization of eosinophils to airway nerves and effect on neuronal M_2 muscarinic receptor function. Am J Physiol 1997; 273(1 Pt 1):L93–L103.
67. Elbon CL, Jacoby DB, Fryer AD. Pretreatment with an antibody to interleukin-5 prevents loss of pulmonary M_2 muscarinic receptor function in antigen challenged guinea-pigs. Am J Respir Cell Mol Biol 1995; 12:320–328.
68. Pretolani M, Ruffie C, Lapa e Silva JR, Joseph D, Lobb RR, Vargaftig BB. Antibody to very late activation antigen 4 prevents antigen-induced bronchial hyperreactivity and cellular infiltration in the guinea pig airways. J Exp Med 1994; 180(3):795–805.
69. Jacoby DB, Gleich GJ, Fryer AD. Human eosinophil major basic protein is an endogenous allosteric antagonist at the inhibitory muscarinic M_2 receptor. J Clin Invest 1993; 91:1314–1318.
70. Walsh JJ, Dietlein LF, Low FN, Burch GE, Mogabgab WJ. Bronchotracheal response in human influenza. Arch Intern Med 1960; 108:376–388.
71. Ada GL, Leung KN, Ertl H. An analysis of effector T cell generation and function in mice exposed to influenza A or Sendai viruses. Immunol Rev 1981; 58:5–24.
72. Samuel CE. Antiviral actions of interferon: interferon-regulated cellular proteins and their surprisingly selective antiviral activities. Virology 1991; 183:1–11.
73. Graham MB, Braciale VL, Braciale TJ. Influenza virus-specific CD4+ T helper type 2 T lymphocytes do not promote recovery from experimental virus infection. J Exp Med 1994; 180(4):1273–1282.
74. Baumgarth N, Brown L, Jackson D, Kelso A. Novel features of the respiratory tract T-cell response to influenza virus infection: lung T cells increase expression of gamma interferon mRNA in vivo and maintain high levels of mRNA expression for interleukin-5 (IL-5) and IL-10. J Virol 1994; 68(11):7575–7581.
75. Coyle AJ, Erard F, Bertrand C, Walti S, Pircher H, Le GG. Virus-specific CD8+ cells can switch to interleukin 5 production and induce airway eosinophilia. J Exp Med 1995; 181(3):1229–1233.
76. Garofalo R, Kimpen JL, Welliver RC, Ogra PL. Eosinophil degranulation in the respiratory tract during naturally acquired respiratory syncytial virus infection. J Pediatr 1992; 120(1):28–32.
77. Openshaw PJ, Clarke SL, Record FM. Pulmonary eosinophilic response to respiratory syncytial virus infection in mice sensitized to the major surface glycoprotein G. Int Immunol 1992; 4(4):493–500.
78. Sigurs N, Bjarnason R, Sigurbergsson F. Eosinophil cationic protein in nasal secretion and in serum and myeloperoxidase in serum in respiratory syncytial

virus bronchiolitis: relation to asthma and atopy. Acta Paediatr 1994; 83(11): 1151–1155.
79. Calhoun WJ, Dick EC, Schwartz LB, Busse WW. A common cold virus, rhinovirus 16, potentiates airway inflammation after segmental antigen bronchoprovocation in allergic subjects. J Clin Invest 1994; 94(6):2200–2208.
80. Frigas E, Loegering DA, Solley GO, Farrow GM, Gleich GJ. Elevated levels of the eosinophil granule MBP in the sputum of patients with bronchial asthma. Mayo Clin Proc 1981; 56:345–353.
81. Adamko DJ, Elwood T, Fryer AD, Jacoby DB. Ovalbumin sensitization changes both the inflammatory response to subsequent viral infection and the mechanism of M_2 muscarinic receptor dysfunction. Am J Respir Crit Care Med 1998; 157: A242.
82. Sorkness R, Clough J, Castleman W, Lemanske RF. Persistent abnormalities in lung physiology and airway parasympathetic conduction after parainfluenza type 1 infection in adult rats. Am Rev Respir Dis 1992; 145:A462.
83. Kahn RN, Okanlami OA, Jacoby DB, Fryer AD. Viral infection induces dependence of neuronal M_2 muscarinic receptors on cyclooxygenase in guinea pig lung. J Clin Invest 1996; 98:299–307.

AUTHOR INDEX

Italicized numbers give the page on which the complete reference is listed.

A

Aas, P, 36, 52, 174, *184*
Abbot, RD, 104, *114*
Abboud, R, 66, 68, *71*, 75, 77, 81, *83*, 166, *169*
Abuan, TH, 81, *85*
Ada, GL, 180, *186*
Adamko, DJ, 181, *187*
Adams, PF, 87, 88, 90, *96*
Adcock, IM, 46, 47, *55*
Addis, GJ, 126, *134*
Aguilina, AT, 104, *113*
Ahmed, B, 79, 81, *84*
Ahmed, T, 15, 20, *26*, 37, *52*, 148, *152*, 174, *184*
Ain-Shoka, AA, 172, *183*
Akaike, T, 173, *184*
Akdis, CA, 104, *113*
Akerlund, A, 106, *115*
al-Nakib, W, 108, 109, *116*, *117*
Alabaster, VA, 17, 27, 41, *54*
Albrecht, JK, 109, *117*
Alessi, DR, 46, *55*
Alexander, J, 103, *113*
Allan, GW, 126, *135*

Allen, SC, 74, 75, *83*
Alleyne, W, 126, *135*
Almquist, JR, 105, *115*
Alroy, G, 126, 129, *133*
Altemus, JB, 4, *22*
Alving, K, 39, *53*
American Thoracic Society, 145, 148, *151*
Anderson, CL, 172, *183*
Anderson, DF, 88, 90, *97*
Ando, M, 173, *184*
Andreis, K, 109, *117*
Angaard, A, 7, 17, 18, *23*, *24*, *28*
Angyard, A, 88, 91, *97*
Ansari, SA, 102, 108, *112*
Anthonisen, NR, 68, *72*, 121, 123, 124, 125, 126, *130*, *131*, *132*, 148, *152*
Antognoni, G, 103, *113*
Aquilina, AT, 171, 173, *183*
Armour, CL, 19, *28*
Arnold, A, 79, 81, *84*
Arrighi, HM, 87, 88, 90, *96*
Arruda, E, 109, *117*
Arthur, J, 104, *114*
Ashe, JH, 34, *51*

189

Ashutosh, K, 66, *71*, 121, 129, *130*, *134*
Atkinson, J, 126, *135*
Attasano, L, 46, *55*
Aubier, M, 121, *131*
Auerbach, D, 147, *151*
Ayala, LE, 15, 20, *26*, 37, *52*, 148, *152*, 174, *184*

B

Bachofen, H, 165, *169*
Badger, GF, 101, 108, *111*, *116*
Ballantyne, A, 160, *168*
Banks, SM, 90, *97*
Bankwala, Z, 63, 69, *70*, 149, *152*
Banov, C, 95, *98*, *99*, 148, *151*, 166, *169*
Bar-Shavit, Z, 177, *185*
Baraniuk, JN, 4, 5, 7, 8, 13, 14, 16, 17, 18, *23*, *24*, *25*, 28, 31, 34, 39, 40, *49*, *53*, 89, 90, 91, *97*
Barclay, J, 126, *134*
Bardin, PG, 103, 109, *112*, *117*
Barnes, PJ, 3, 4, 5, 6, 7, 8, 13, 14, 15, 16, 17, 18, 19, 20, *22*, *23*, *24*, *25*, *26*, *27*, *28*, 29, 31, 32, 33, 34, 35, 36, 37, 39, 40, 41, 42, 43, 44, 45, 46, 47, 48, 49, *49*, *50*, *51*, *52*, *53*, *54*, *55*, 59, 61, 63, 64, *69*, *70*, 120, 122, 124, *130*, *132*, 137, 139, 140, 141, 142, 143, 144, 145, 148, 149, *150*, *152*, 166, 167, *169*, 174, *184*
Baroody, FM, 91, 93, *98*
Barros, MJ, 126, *134*
Barrow, GI, 108, 109, *116*, *117*
Barrow, I, 104, *114*
Basbaum, CB, 7, *24*, 32, *49*, 59, *69*, 90, *97*, 122, 124, *132*
Baskerville, J, 126, 127, *135*
Bassett, DJP, 15, *27*
Bassow, L, 106, *115*
Bateman, RJM, 69, *72*
Baton, CA, 90, *97*

Battista, C, 87, 88, 90, *96*
Batty, IH, 15, *27*
Bauman, KA, 102, *111*
Baumgartener-Folkerts, C, 34, *51*
Baumgarth, N, 180, *186*
Baumgartner, C, 14, *25*, 33, *50*
Bayston, S, 79, 81, *84*
Beakes, De, 166, *169*
Beasley, PP, 104, *114*
Beck, KC, 14, *25*
Beck, MA, 172, *183*
Beck, R, 81, *85*
Becker, AB, 74, 75, *83*
Becker, B, 107, *116*
Becker, EL, 177, *185*
Becker, S, 172, *183*
Beld, AJ, 7, 14, 19, *24*, *28*, 32, *50*
Bell, G, 129, *134*
Belman, MJ, 129, *133*
Belton, PA, 160, *168*
Belvisi, MG, 4, 5, 7, 15, 19, *23*, *26*, *28*, 36, 40, 41, 42, *52*, *54*, 137, 140, 141, *150*
Bender, BS, 172, *183*
Benson, V, 102, *111*
Berend, N, 126, 127, *135*
Berg, O, 108, *116*
Berger, R, 129, *134*
Berkowitz, RB, 106, *115*
Bernedo, P, 32, 34, *50*
Bernstein, A, 75, 77, 81, *83*
Berrie, CP, 33, *50*
Berry, RB, 129, *134*
Bertley, JC, 124, *132*
Bertrand, C, 180, *186*
Betermann, J, 14, *25*
Beumer, HM, 128, *133*
Biondi, R, 95, *99*
Birdsall, NJM, 31, 33, *49*, *50*
Bjarnason, R, 180, *186*
Blaber, LC, 36, *52*, 174, *184*
Black, JL, 19, *28*
Blank, MA, 7, *23*
Blankenstieijn, WM, 32, *50*

Blankesteijn, WM, 7, 14, *24*
Blaser, K, 104, *113*
Bleecker, E, 127, *136*
Bleecker, ER, 121, 128, *130*, *133*
Bleeker, E, 65, 66, *71*
Blennerhassett, G, 66, *71*, 126, 127, *135*
Bloom, JW, 14, 16, 17, *25*, 32, 33, 34, *50*, *51*
Bluestone, CD, 106, *115*
Boat, TF, 90, *97*
Boe, J, 77, *84*
Bogaert, M, 121, *131*
Boggs, P, 95, *99*, 148, *151*, 166, *169*
Boggs, PB, 95, *98*
Boner, AL, 81, *85*
Bonetti, S, 81, *85*
Bonizzato, C, 81, *85*
Bonner, TI, 8, *24*
Borman, G, 77, *84*
Borson, DB, 172, 177, *183*
Borum, P, 18, *28*, 107, *116*
Botnick, WC, 129, *133*
Boulan, ER, 176, *185*
Boushey, HA, 18, *28*, 129, *134*
Bovbjerg, DH, 103, *113*
Bowen, RE, 64, *71*
Bowie, DM, 149, *152*
Braciale, TJ, 180, *186*
Braciale, VL, 180, *186*
Brandon, B, 106, *115*
Brann, MR, 8, *24*, 40, *54*
Branum, JP, 129, *134*
Braun, S, 122, 127, *132*, *136*
Braun, SR, 121, *130*
Brewis, RAL, 160, *168*
Brezina, I, 90, *97*
British Thoracic Society, 73, 81, *82*
Britt, EJ, 128, *133*
Brochard, L, 74, *83*
Broderick, DJ, 176, *185*
Bronsky, E, 94, 95, *98*, *99*, 148, *151*
Bronsky, EA, 95, *98*, 148, *151*
Brophy, C, 79, 81, *84*

Brown, IG, 126, *135*
Brown, JG, 126, *134*
Brown, JR, 33, *50*
Brown, L, 180, *186*
Brown, R, 46, *55*
Bruinvels, A, 10, *25*
Bryant, D, 75, 77, *83*
Buckley, CM, 8, *24*
Buckley, NJ, 8, 17, *24*, *27*, 31, 35, 40, 42, *49*, *51*, *54*
Buckner, CK, 172, 173, *183*, *184*
Buick, B, 121, *131*
Buist, AS, 77, *84*
Burch, GE, 179, *186*
Burchfiel, CM, 103, *113*
Burgen, AS, 33, *50*
Burns, JJ, 104, *114*
Burrell, CJ, 104, 105, *113*
Busse, WW, 171, 172, 173, 180, *182*, *183*, *184*, *187*

C

Calhoun, WJ, 180, *187*
Caliguiri, LA, 176, *185*
Callahan, S, 66, *71*, 79, 81, *84*
Callahan, W, 148, *151*
Calvarese, B, 129, *134*
Calverley, PMA, 121, *130*
Campbell, AH, 74, *83*
Campbell, S, 147, *151*
Canny, G, 66, *71*, 79, 81, *84*, *85*, 148, *151*
Cantekin, EL, 106, *115*
Caputi, M, 126, 127, *135*
Carenfelt, C, 108, *116*
Carer, J, 63, *71*
Carilli, AD, 171, *182*
Carisson, LG, 77, *84*
Carroll, R, 11, *25*
Casale, TB, 20, *29*, 32, 34, *50*, 122, *132*
Castaneda, C, 158, *168*
Castleman, W, 181, *187*

Castleman, WL, 176, *185*
Cate, TR, 103, *112*
Cattarossi, L, 7, *24*
Caulfield, MP, 3, 5, 6, 8, 11, 14, 15, 16, 18, *22*
Cazzola, M, 33, *50*, 126, 127, *135*
Cecchin, A, 109, *117*
Celli, BR, 122, *132*
Challiss, RAI, 3, 8, 11, 15, 16, 18, *22*
Challiss, RAJ, 39, *53*
Chambers, DK, 75, 77, 81, *83*
Chan, CS, 126, *134*, *135*
Chan-Li, Y, 178, 179, *186*
Chang, EM, 126, *134*
Chapman, KR, 66, 68, 69, *71*, *72*, 75, 77, 81, *83*, 127, 129, *134*, 137, 145, 148, 149, *150*, *152*, 156, 160, 165, 166, *167*, *169*
Chau, LK, 124, *132*
Cheong, B, 74, *83*
Cherniack, RM, 67, *71*, 148, *151*
Chervinsky, P, 95, *99*
Chiari, MC, 40, *54*
Chilvers, ER, 15, *27*, 39, *53*
Chiplunkar, R, 122, *132*
Choi, AMK, 172, 173, *183*, *184*
Choppin, PW, 176, *185*
Chow, S, 35, 39, *51*
Chow, SP, 11, 20, *25*, *29*
Chuange, D, 44, *55*
Clancy, J, 40, *53*
Clapham, D, 11, *25*
Clark, JR, 102, 108, *112*
Clark, RA, 123, 127, *132*
Clark, TJH, 74, *83*
Clarke, SL, 180, *186*
Clarke, SW, 69, *72*
Claverley, PMA, 122, *131*
Clayton, DE, 172, *183*
Clough, J, 181, *187*
Clough, JJ, 176, *185*
Clyde, WA, 171, *182*
Co, E, 60, *70*
Cobb, MH, 46, *55*

Coburn, RF, 4, *22*
Coe, C, 42, *54*
Coe, CI, 166, *169*
Coffman, TM, 172, *183*
Cogswell, JI, 103, *113*
Cohen, M, 171, *182*
Cohen, P, 46, *55*
Cohen, S, 103, *113*
Cohen, SG, 161, *168*
Colasurdo, GN, 172, *183*
Coles, SJ, 7, *23*
Collier, AM, 171, *182*
Colonno, RJ, 110, *117*
Combivent Inhalational Aerosol Study Group, 126, *135*
Compans, RW, 176, *185*
Connett, JE, 68, *72*, 77, *84*, 121, 125, *130*, 148, *152*
Connolly, CK, 40, *54*
Cook, D, 122, 124, *132*
Cook, DN, 172, *183*
Corne, JM, 81, *84*
Cornelissen, PJ, 63, *70*
Cornelissen, PJG, 42, *54*, 127, 128, *133*, *136*, 145, 146, 147, 149, *151*
Coroneos, E, 48, *55*
Corrado, A, 124, 129, *133*
Costello, RW, 15, *26*, 39, *52*, *53*, 174, 176, 178, 179, *184*, *186*
Costongs, MAL, 42, *54*, 145, *151*
Couch, RB, 103, 109, *112*, *117*
Coyle, AJ, 180, *186*
Crump, CE, 109, *117*
Cuenda, A, 46, *55*
Curtis, CAM, 10, *25*
Cusack, TM, 102, 108, *112*
Cuss, FM, 15, *27*, 33, *50*

D

D'Agostino, G, 15, 20, *26*, 40, *54*
Dale, HH, 8, *24*
Dales, RE, 68, *72*, 127, 129, *134*
Davies, D, 75, 77, *83*, *84*, 129, *134*

Davies, L, 104, 105, *113*
Davison, I, 122, *131*
de Santis, D, 33, *50*
De Zeeuw, RA, 35, *51*, 127, 129, *133*
Dean, HG, 42, *54*
Debaker-Williame, E, 171, *182*
Debelle, P, 104, 105, *113*
Decramer, M, 148, *151*
Delwiche, JP, 124, 126, *133*
DeMeo, AN, 171, *182*
Dent, AG, 126, *134*, *135*
Dent, G, 121, *131*
Desa, MM, 129, *134*
Dessanges, JF, 18, *28*
DeStafano, G, 81, *85*
Dev, G, 129, *134*
Dev, RD, 7, *23*
Devillier, P, 18, *28*
Dey, R, 4, *22*
Dhillon, DP, 123, 127, *132*
Dhingra, S, 123, 126, *132*
Diamant, Z, 15, *27*
Diamond, L, 107, 108, *116*, 148, *151*
Dick, EC, 103, 110, *112*, *117*, 171, 172, 173, 180, *182*, *183*, *184*, *187*
Dickinson, G, 68, *72*, 127, 129, *134*
Dietlein, LF, 179, *186*
Dingle, JH, 101, 108, *111*, *116*
Disse, B, 41, 42, 43, *54*, 137, 139, 140, 141, *150*
Dixon, CMS, 15, 20, *26*, 37, *52*, 148, *152*, 174, *184*
Djokic, TD, 172, *183*
Dockhorn, R, 95, *99*, 107, *116*
Dockhorn, RJ, 107, *116*, 148, *151*
Dolorich, J, 93, *98*
Dolovich, J, 66, *71*
Donohue, JF, 122, *131*
Dorje, F, 8, *24*, 40, *54*
Douglas, NJ, 122, *131*, 149, *152*
Douglas, R, 103, *112*
Douglas, RG, 104, *113*, 171, 173, *182*, *183*
Douglas, RM, 104, 105, 109, *113*, *117*

Doyle, WJ, 104, *113*
Driesner, NK, 81, *85*
Druce, H, 95, *98*, 148, *151*
Druce, HM, 18, *28*, 88, 90, 91, *91*, *95*, 97, *97*, *98*
Dubois, PEP, 124, 126, *133*
Dudley, DT, 46, *55*
Duerson, K, 11, *25*
Dullinger, D, 121, *131*
Duncan, C, 123, 126, *132*
Dunn, L, 147, *151*
Dusser, DJ, 172, *183*
Duvoisin, RC, 157, *168*
Dykes, MH, 104, *114*

E

Eadie, MB, 171, *182*
Earis, JE, 121, 122, *130*, *131*
Easton, PA, 121, 123, 126, *131*, *132*
Eberlein, RS, 73, *82*
Eby, GA, 105, *114*
Ecklund, P, 32, 34, *50*
Edmonson, WP, 103, *112*
Eggleston, PA, 104, 105, *113*
Eglen, RM, 3, 8, 10, 11, 15, 16, 18, *22*, *24*, 35, 39, *51*
Ehlert, FJ, 15, *26*
Eigen, H, 108, *116*
Einarsson, O, 173, *183*
El Sanadi, N, 79, *84*
El-Fakahany, EE, 176, *185*
Elad, Y, 104, *114*
Elbon, CL, 15, *26*, 36, 38, 39, *51*, *52*, *53*, 178, *185*, *186*
Elias, JA, 173, *183*
Eller, JJ, 171, *182*
Elliott, HL, 165, *169*
Ellis, DA, 127, 129, *134*
Ellis, EF, 171, *182*
Ellis, MH, 108, *116*
Elwood, T, 177, 181, *185*, *187*
Elzinga, CRS, 35, 39, *51*, *53*
Emala, CW, 40, *53*

Emmick, G, 81, *85*
Empey, DW, 104, *113*, 171, 173, 174, *182*
Engelstatter, R, 33, *50*
English, JA, 102, *111*
Enright, PL, 77, *84*
Erard, F, 180, *186*
Ernsberger, P, 7, *24*
Ernst, E, 105, *114*
Ernst, P, 78, *84*
Ertl, H, 180, *186*
Ervenius, O, 165, *169*
Evans, CM, 15, *26*, 39, *53*, 174, 179, *184*

F

Fahrenkrug, J, 7, 17, *23*
Fakahany, EE, 38, *52*
Fanta, C, 75, 81, *84, 85*
Fanta, CH, 77, *84*
Farah, A, 121, *131*
Farr, BM, 108, 110, *116, 117*
Farrow, GM, 180, *187*
Faulkner, D, 36, *51*
Felder, CC, 13, 16, *25*
Feldman, W, 102, 106, *111*
Fentem, PH, 75, *83*, 129, *134*
Ferguson, GT, 67, *71*
Fergusson, DM, 103, *113*
Fernandes, LB, 19, 20, *29*, 35, *51*
Fernandez, R, 149, *152*
Filuk, RB, 121, *131*
Findlay, S, 148, *151*
Findlay, SR, 95, *98*, 148, *151*
Fink, G, 129, *134*
Finn, A, 95, *99*
Fireman, P, 93, 95, *98*, 106, *115*
Fischer, A, 4, *23*
Fitzgerald, JD, 64, *71*, 129, *134*
Fitzgerald, JM, 75, 76, 77, 78, 81, *84*
Flatley, M, 127, *136*
Flavahan, NA, 14, *25*
Flenley, DC, 122, *131*

Fong, J, 33, *50*
Ford, M, 177, *185*
Ford, S, 93, *98*
Forstall, GJ, 104, *114*
Forsyth, BR, 171, *182*
Forts, D, 148, *151*
Fothergill, JM, 163, *168*
Fox, AJ, 42, *54*
Fraenkel, D, 103, *112*
Frankel, A, 77, *84*
Franzuso, G, 46, *55*
Fraser, CM, 10, 11, 12, *24, 25*
Freidman, M, 122, *131*
Frick, OK, 171, 173, *182*
Frick, WE, 171, *182*
Friedman, M, 68, *72*, 121, 124, *130*, 147, 149, *151, 152*
Frigas, E, 180, *187*
Frith, PA, 126, *135*
Fryer, A, 15, *27*, 175, 176, 179, 181, *185, 187*
Fryer, AD, 15, 19, 20, 21, *26, 27*, 29, 35, 36, 38, 39, 40, *51, 52, 53*, 148, *152*, 174, 177, 178, 179, 181, *184, 185, 186, 187*
Fukamauchi, F, 44, *55*
Fulginiti, VA, 171, *182*
Fuller, RW, 37, *52*
Furguson, GT, 148, *151*

G

Gabbay, U, 129, *134*
Gadomski, A, 107, *116*
Gaffey, MJ, 106, 109, *115*
Gaitini, L, 126, 129, *133*
Galant, SP, 17, *27*
Galdes-Sebalt, M, 81, *85*
Gambone, LM, 39, *53*
Gandevia, B, 137, *150*, 160, 163, *168*
Garofalo, R, 180, *186*
Garrett, J, 77, 81, *84, 85*
Garrett, JE, 75, 76, 77, 78, 80, 81, 82, *84*, 148, *151*

Gelb, A, 74, *83*
Gent, M, 166, *169*
Gentry, E, 63, 68, *70*, 123, 126, *132*
Georgitis, J, 95, *99*, 148, *151*
Georgitis, JW, 95, *98*, 148, *151*
German, DF, 171, 173, *182*
Getz, M, 66, *71*
Ghaem, A, 18, *28*
Ghafouri, M, 68, *72*, 121, 124, *130*
Giacopelli, A, 127, 128, *133*
Gibson, GJ, 124, *133*
Gibson, J, 148, *151*
Giembycz, MA, 20, *29*, 44, 45, *55*
Gies, J, 38, *52*
Gies, JP, 15, *26*, 176, *185*
Ginneken, CAM, 17, *28*
Gleich, GJ, 15, 21, *26*, 27, *29*, 39, *52*, *53*, 174, 178, 179, 180, *184*, *186*, *187*
Glezen, WP, 103, *112*
Godfrey, JC, 105, *114*
Godfrey, JM, 105, *114*
Gohd, RS, 171, *182*
Gold, WM, 17, *27*, 171, 173, 174, *182*
Golde, DW, 48, *55*
Goldie, RG, 172, *183*
Goldman, R, 177, *185*
Goldsmith, EJ, 46, *55*
Gomm, SA, 74, 75, *83*
Goodman, DL, 64, *71*
Gordon, W, 171, *182*
Gorini, M, 124, 129, *133*
Goswami, SK, 7, 11, *23*
Gottfried, SB, 124, *132*
Gourlay, HS, 127, *136*
Gowdy, JM, 157, 160, *168*
Graham, MB, 180, *186*
Graham, NM, 104, 105, *113*
Grana, E, 40, *54*
Grandordy, B, 19, *28*
Grandordy, BM, 15, *27*, 33, *50*
Graninger, W, 33, *50*
Graves, JP, 172, *183*
Graves, R, 157, *168*

Green, BQ, 106, *115*
Green, S, 42, *54*
Greenberg, D, 63, 68, *70*, 123, 126, *132*
Greenberg, SB, 109, *117*
Greenstone, M, 79, 81, *84*
Grieco, MH, 65, *71*
Griffin, MT, 15, *26*
Grist, NR, 171, *182*
Gross, NJ, 60, 61, 63, 64, 66, 67, 69, *70*, *71*, 75, *83*, 122, 126, *131*, *132*, 137, 145, 148, 149, *150*, *152*, 167, *169*
Grossman, J, 93, 95, *98*, *99*, 107, *116*, 148, *151*, 166, *169*
Guerra, F, 159, *168*
Gump, DW, 171, *182*
Gupta, GL, 60, *70*
Gutersohn, J, 126, *135*
Guyatt, GH, 122, 124, *132*
Guyer, B, 102, 108, *112*
Gwaltney, J, 102, *111*
Gwaltney, JM, 101, 103, 104, 105, 106, 108, 109, 110, *111*, *112*, *113*, *115*, *116*, *117*

H

Hacksell, U, 10, *25*
Haddad, E, 35, 39, 40, 41, 43, *51*, *53*, *54*, 137, 139, 141, *150*
Haddad, EB, 15, 17, 19, 20, *26*, *27*, *28*, *29*, 39, 44, 45, 46, 47, 48, *53*, *55*
Haddad, el-B, 49, *55*
Haddox, R, 127, *136*
Halayko, AJ, 120, *130*
Hall, WJ, 104, *113*, 171, 173, *182*, *183*
Halonen, M, 14, 16, 17, *25*, 32, 33, 34, *50*, *51*
Halsey, TJ, 15, *27*
Hamamoto, T, 173, *184*
Hammer, R, 33, 41, 42, 43, *50*, *54*, 137, 139, 140, 141, *150*

Hampel, FC, 148, *151*
Hamstra, JJ, 21, *29*
Hargreave, FE, 66, *71*
Harlow, ES, 165, *169*
Harrington, C, 42, *54*
Harris, JM, 103, *112*
Harrison, AC, 126, 127, *135*
Haslett, C, 129, *134*
Hauptschein-Raphael, M, 93, *98*
Haxhiu, MA, 7, *24*
Haxhiu-Poskurica, B, 7, *24*
Hay, JG, 63, *71*
Hayden, FB, 110, *117*
Hayden, FG, 101, 105, 106, 108, 109, *111*, *114*, *115*, *116*, *117*, 148, *151*
Hayes, VY, 15, *27*
Haynes, RL, 63, *70*
Heath, RB, 177, *185*
Heffner, J, 122, *132*
Hegde, SS, 8, 10, 16, *24*, 35, 39, *51*
Heinz-Erian, P, 7, *23*
Hemila, H, 104, *114*
Hemming, VG, 172, *183*
Hendeles, L, 106, *115*
Henderson, FW, 171, 172, *182*, *183*
Hendley, JO, 101, 103, 104, 105, 108, 110, *111*, *112*, *113*, *114*, *116*, *117*
Henry, PJ, 172, *183*
Hermanussen, MW, 7, *24*
Hertz, CW, 162, 164, *168*
Hervonen, A, 7, *23*
Herxheimer, H, 165, *169*
Herzog, H, 126, *135*
Hetta, L, 77, *84*
Hey, C, 15, *26*
Hibert, MF, 10, *25*
Higgenbottom, T, 148, *151*
Higgins, MW, 103, *113*
Higgins, PG, 108, 109, *116*, *117*
Higgins, RM, 75, *83*
Hightower, CE, 156, 158, *167*
Hill, JS, 88, *97*
Hirano, T, 173, *184*

Hirschman, CA, 19, 20, *29*, 35, *51*
Hirschowitz, BI, 33, *50*
Hirshman, CA, 40, *53*
Hoffman, EA, 122, *132*
Hoffman, LS, 171, *182*
Hoflack, J, 10, *25*
Hokfelt, T, 6, *23*
Holgafe, ST, 88, 90, *97*
Holgate, ST, 81, *84*, 108, *116*, 126, *135*
Holmstedt, B, 165, *169*
Holt, E, 102, 108, *112*
Hopkin, JM, 127, 129, *134*
Horsley, MG, 75, 77, 81, *83*
Horton, L, 107, *116*
Horwood, LJ, 103, *113*
Hosey, MM, 10, 11, 12, 13, 14, 16, *25*
Hossain, SU, 110, *117*
Hough, C, 44, *55*
Howard, P, 148, *151*
Howarth, PH, 126, *135*
Huang, YC, 176, 179, *185*
Hudgel, D, 149, *152*
Hudgel, DW, 81, *85*
Hueston, WJ, , 102, 108, *112*
Hughart, N, 102, 108, *112*
Huhti, E, 126, *135*
Hulme, EC, 31, 33, *49*, *50*
Hume, KM, 166, *169*
Hummel, AM, 15, *27*
Hurd, J, 177, *185*
Hutton, N, 106, *115*

I

Igarashi, Y, 104, 105, *113*
Ikeda, A, 62, 63, *70*, *71*, 123, 126, 128, 129, *132*, *133*, *134*
Illowite, J, 147, *151*
Ind, PW, 37, *52*
Ingram, CG, 126, 127, *135*
Ingram, RH, 63, *70*

International Rhinitis Management
 Working Group, 88, *96*
Ishihara, H, 14, 16, *25*
Ito, Y, 36, *52*, 174, *184*
Izumi, T, 62, 63, *70*, *71*, 123, 126,
 128, 129, *132*, *133*, *134*

J

Jackson, CM, 123, 127, *132*
Jackson, D, 180, *186*
Jackson, JL, 105, *114*
Jackson, RT, 93, *98*
Jacobs, L, 104, *113*, 171, 173, 174,
 182
Jacobsen, H, 102, 108, *112*
Jacoby, D, 181, *187*
Jacoby, DB, 15, 20, 21, *26*, *27*, *29*,
 36, 38, 39, *51*, *52*, *53*, 172, 173,
 174, 175, 176, 177, 178, 179, 181,
 183, *184*, *185*, *186*, *187*
Jadue, C, 123, 126, *132*
Jaeschke, R, 122, 124, *132*
Jain, DK, 60, *70*
Jalowayski, AA, 89, 90, *97*
Janowski, R, 93, *98*
Janson, C, 77, *84*
Janssen, PA, 109, *117*
Januskiewicz, A, 104, *114*
Jarvis, D, 7, *23*
Jarvis, MJ, 103, *113*
Jenne, JW, 121, *131*
Jenner, B, 126, *135*
Jennings, LC, 103, *112*
Johnson, CE, 156, 158, *167*
Johnson, DW, 66, *71*, 79, 81, *84*, 148,
 151
Johnson, LR, 77, *84*
Johnson, PA, 68, *72*, 121, 124, *130*
Johnston, RN, 126, 127, *135*
Johnston, S, 81, *84*
Johnston, SL, 103, 108, 109, *112*, *116*,
 117, 171, 172, *182*

Jones, BMJ, 74, *83*
Jones, CA, 33, *50*
Jones, NL, 149, *152*
Jonsson, L, 91, *97*
Joos, H, 126, *135*
Jordan, WS, 101, 108, *111*, *116*
Jorres, RA, 121, 129, *131*
Joseph, D, 178, *186*
Jubarin, A, 126, 129, *133*
Julia-Serda, G, 18, *28*

K

Kabela, E, 121, *131*
Kagey-Sobotka, A, 93, *98*
Kahn, R, 181, *187*
Kaik, G, 126, *135*
Kailis, SG, 121, *131*
Kaiser, DL, 63, *70*, 106, 109, 110,
 115, *117*
Kaiser, H, 148, *151*
Kaliner, M, 90, 93, *97*, *98*
Kaliner, MA, 7, 8, 13, 14, 16, 17, 18,
 23, *24*, *28*, 39, *53*, 90, 91, *97*
Kalishker, A, 149, *152*
Kaminski, D, 124, *133*
Kane, FJ, 106, *115*
Kanjanapothi, D, 160, *168*
Karen, DL, 106, *115*
Karlson, B, 77, *84*
Karpel, JP, 63, 68, *70*, 75, 76, 77, 81,
 84, 123, 126, *132*, *135*
Kasel, JA, 103, *112*
Kawakatsu, K, 129, *133*
Kaye, C, 129, *134*
Kazim, F, 81, *85*
Keller, JB, 103, *113*
Kelly, AM, 75, 77, 78, 80, 81, 82, *84*,
 148, *151*
Kelly, CA, 126, *134*, *135*
Kelso, A, 180, *186*
Kephart, GM, 15, *26*, 39, *52*, 178,
 186

Kester, M, 48, *55*
Khawaja, AM, 39, *53*
Kilbinger, H, 17, *27*, 40, *54*
Kiley, JF, 148, *152*
Kiley, JP, 68, *72*, 121, 125, *130*
Kilibinger, H, 15, 20, *26*
Killian, KJ, 149, *152*
Kim, AL, 36, *51*, 178, *185*
Kimpen, JL, 180, *186*
Kinney, C, 121, *131*
Kirschstein, RL, 177, *185*
Kirsten, DK, 121, 129, *131*
Kisicki, JC, 148, *151*
Klapproth, H, 32, 34, *50*
Klassen, ABM, 7, 14, 17, *24*, 28, 32, *50*
Kleinerman, JI, 90, *97*
Klint, T, 106, *115*
Knobil, K, 173, *184*
Koesling, D, 4, *23*
Koeter, GH, 127, 129, *133*
Kogan, MD, 102, *111*
Koker, P, 148, *151*
Kolesnick, R, 48, *55*
Koling, A, 91, *97*
Konig, P, 108, *116*
Korenblatt, P, 95, *99*
Korts, D, 148, *151*
Korts, DC, 108, *116*
Kossoff, D, 18, *28*, 91, *97*
Koster, F, 102, *111*
Kotch, A, 126, *135*
Kotelchuck, M, 102, *111*
Kowal, MB, 63, *70*
Koyama, H, 62, 63, *70, 71*, 123, 126, 128, 129, *132, 133, 134*
Kradjan, WA, 81, *85*
Kreisman, H, 75, 77, 81, *83*
Krikke, M, 38, *52*
Krivoy, N, 126, 129, *133*
Kronenberg, R, 121, *131*
Kubo, T, 14, *25*
Kummer, W, 4, *23*
Kuo, H, 32, *49*

Kuo, HP, 15, *27*
Kurian, SS, 7, *23*
Kurtenbach, E, 10, *25*

L

Lacroix, JS, 7, 18, *24*, 39, *53*
Lagnner, A, 33, *50*
Laitinen, A, 7, *23*
Laitinen, LA, 7, *23*, 104, *113*, 171, 173, 174, *182*
Lakkis, H, 81, *85*
Laliberte, G, 68, *72*, 127, 129, *134*
Lamborn, KR, 171, *182*
Lambrecht, G, 8, *24*
Lammers, J, 37, *52*, 148, *152*
Lammers, JW, 4, *23*
Lammers, JWJ, 7, 14, 19, *24, 25*, 28, 34, *50*, 174, *184*
Lamont, H, 121, *131*
Lamy, ME, 171, *182*
Landau, LI, 66, *71*
Landry, Y, 38, *52*, 176, *185*
Lane, DJ, 75, *83*
Lanes, S, 77, *84*
Lanes, SF, 76, 77, 81, *84*
Lang, RE, 4, *23*
Langston, L, 81, *85*
Lanners, J, 15, 20, *26*
Lapa e Silva, JR, 178, *186*
Larsen, GL, 172, *183*
Lathotia, M, 60, *70*
Laughlin, KR, 126, 127, *135*
Lawford, P, 74, *83*
Lawrence, LJ, 32, 34, *50*
Lawson, KA, 87, 88, 90, *96*
Lazareno, S, 40, *54*
Le, GG, 180, *186*
Lea, P, 106, *115*
Leahy, B, 74, 75, *83*
LeBlanc, P, 149, *152*
LeDoux, EJ, 123, 126, *132*
Lee, NH, 10, 11, 12, *24*, 178, 179, *186*

Leenen, FH, 165, *169*
Leenen, FHH, 69, *72*, 149, *152*
Lees, AW, 126, *135*
Lefcoe, NM, 66, *71*, 126, 127, *135*
Legge, JS, 126, 127, *135*
Leitch, AG, 127, 129, *134*
Lemanske, RF, 171, 176, 181, *182*, *185*, *187*
Lesko, E, 105, *114*
Leung, KN, 180, *186*
Levey, AI, 36, 40, *51*, *54*, 178, *185*
Levin, DC, 126, 127, *135*
Levine, PA, 101, 109, *111*, *117*
Levine, SJ, 120, *130*
Levinson, H, 66, *71*
Levison, H, 79, 81, *84*, *85*, 148, *151*
Levy, SF, 121, 122, 124, *130*, *132*
Lewis, D, 149, *152*
Lichtenstein, LM, 93, *98*, 103, 104, *112*
Light, RW, 129, *134*
Lightboy, IM, 126, 127, *135*
Lin, TY, 73, *82*
Lin, X, 4, *23*
Lindsay, MA, 46, 47, 48, 49, *55*
Lippiet, P, 160, *168*
Lipworth, BJ, 123, 127, *132*
Little, JW, 171, 173, *182*
Little, KS, 126, 127, *135*
Littner, M, 147, *151*
Ljungholm, K, 77, *84*
Lloberes, P, 123, 127, 128, *132*
Loader, JE, 172, *183*
Lobb, RR, 178, *186*
Lockhart, A, 18, *28*
Loegering, DA, 180, *187*
Logun, C, 14, 16, 17, *25*, 90, *97*
Longini, IM, 110, *117*
Lotvall, J, 164, *168*
Low, FN, 179, *186*
Lowenstein,SR, 106, *115*
Lowry, RC, 121, *131*
Luciani, G, 127, 128, *133*
Lulling, J, 124, 126, *133*

Lumry, W, 95, *99*
Lundberg, JM, 7, 17, 18, *23*, *24*, *28*, 39, *53*
Lundblad, L, 18, *28*
Lundgren, JD, 90, 92, 93, *97*
Luparello, T, 65, *71*
Luursema, PB, 128, *133*
Lybass,TG, 171, *182*
Lyons, HA, 65, *71*

M

Macfarlane, JT, 77, *84*, 129, *134*
MacGregor, T, 93, *98*
Machlin, LJ, 104, *114*
Mackenzie, JS, 172, *183*
Macknin, M, 105, *114*
Macknin, ML, 104, *114*
Maclagan, J, 15, 20, *26*, 31, 33, 36, 40, *49*, *51*, *52*, 174, *184*
Madison, JM, 33, *50*
Maeda, A, 14, *25*
Maeda, H, 173, *184*
Maesen, FP, 63, *70*
Maesen, FPV, 42, *54*, 145, 146, 147, 149, *151*
Magnussen, H, 19, *28*, 35, *51*, 121, 129, *131*
Mahler, DA, 121, *131*
Mainous, AG, 102, 108, *112*
Mak, JC, 15, *27*, 39, *53*
Mak, JCW, 7, 13, 14, 16, 17, 19, 20, *24*, *27*, *28*, *29*, 31, 32, 34, 35, 39, 40, 41, 44, 45, 46, 47, *49*, *50*, *51*, *54*, *55*, 137, 139, 141, *150*
Mal, H, 74, *83*
Malone, DC, 87, 88, 90, *96*
Maltais, F, 124, *132*
Mandel, EM, 106, *115*
Marano, MA, 87, 88, 90, *96*, 102, *111*
Marasco, Wa, 177, *185*
Marci, F, 103, *113*
Marcus, HI, 65, *71*, 166, *169*
Marderosian, AH, 156, *167*

Marlin, GE, 126, 127, *135*
Marlin, SD, 109, *117*
Marmo, E, 33, *50*
Marom, Z, 7, 11, *23*, 90, *97*
Martin, RJ, 7, *24*, 149, *152*
Martinez, FD, 103, *113*
Martling, C, 39, *53*
Massague, J, 46, *55*
Matera, MG, 126, 127, *135*
Mathew, S, 104, *114*
Matran, R, 39, *53*
Mavoungov, E, 15, *27*
Mayer, B, 4, 22, *23*
Mazur, JE, 73, *82*
McCaffrey, TV, 17, *28*
McCormack, DG, 15, *27*, 39, *53*
McCusker, M, 4, 14, *23*, 25, 34, *50*
McCusker, MT, 15, 20, *26*, 37, *52*, 148, *152*, 174, *184*
McDevitt, DG, 121, *131*
McDonald, DM, 172, *183*
McFadden, ER, 63, 65, *70*, 71, 77, 79, 81, *84*, *85*, 160, *168*
McGivern, D, 79, 81, *84*
McHardy, GJR, 127, 129, *134*
McIntosh, K, 81, *85*, 171, *182*
Mead, J, 63, *70*
Medendorp, SV, 104, 105, *114*
Mehta, S, 60, *70*
Meier, P, 104, *114*
Mellits, ED, 106, *115*
Meltzer, E, 94, *98*, 148, *151*
Meltzer, EO, 88, 89, 90, 94, 95, *96*, *97*, *98*, *99*, 102, *111*
Mendez, R, 121, *131*
Menjoge, S, 147, *151*
Merchant, S, 127, 129, *134*
Meredith, SD, 90, *97*
Merida, M, 7, 8, 13, 14, 16, 17, *24*
Merus, H, 7, 21, *24*, *29*
Merus, M, 35, *51*
Meryn, S, 33, *50*
Meurs, H, 31, *49*
Middleton, E, 149, *152*

Midorikawa, J, 37, *52*, 174, *184*
Miles, HB, 109, *117*
Milgrom, H, 95, *99*
Milledge, JS, 74, *83*
Miller, MJ, 7, *24*
Miller, RD, 108, *116*
Mills, J, 171, 173, *182*
Minette, M, 4, *23*
Minette, P, 14, 15, *25*, *27*, 34, 39, *50*, *53*, 124, 126, *133*, 174, *184*
Minette, PA, 15, 20, *26*, 31, 36, *49*, *51*
Minette, PAH, 37, *52*, 148, *152*
Mink, KA, 103, 110, *112*, *117*
Minor, TE, 171, *182*
Mishima, M, 129, *134*
Mishina, M, 14, *25*
Misuri, G, 124, 129, *133*
Mitchell, EB, 103, *113*
Moerman, E, 121, *131*
Mogabgab, WJ, 179, *186*
Molfino, NA, 18, *28*
Molina, E, 33, *50*
Molkenboer, JFWM, 127, *136*
Monto, AS, 110, *117*
Montserrat, JM, 123, 127, 128, *132*
Moore, BW, 109, *117*
Morgan, A, 129, *134*
Morikawa, M, 172, *183*
Morris, JF, 123, 126, *132*
Morrison, BJ, 103, *113*
Morrison, JFJ, 42, *54*
Morton, O, 128, *133*
Mossad, SB, 105, *114*
Mossberg, B, 77, *84*
Mostert, R, 127, *136*
Mudholkar, GS, 171, 173, *182*
Mukherjec, J, 93, *98*
Mulder, J, 81, *85*
Mullarkey, MF, 88, *97*
Mullol, J, 14, 16, 17, *25*, 39, *53*, 90, 92, 93, *97*
Murray, AB, 103, *113*
Mutschler, E, 8, *24*

Mygind, N, 18, *28*, 88, 91, *97*, 103, 107, *112*, *116*

N

Nacleno, R, 93, *98*
Naclerio, RM, 88, 89, 91, 93, *97*, *98*, 103, 104, *112*
Nadel, JA, 7, *24*, 32, *49*, 59, 60, *69*, 90, *97*, 122, 124, *132*, 171, 172, 173, 174, 177, *182*, *183*
Nahorski, SR, 15, *27*, 39, *53*
Nakazawa, H, 172, *183*
Naline, E, 15, *27*
Nanavati, S, 10, *25*
Nathan, RA, 88, *96*
Neale, JM, 103, *113*
Nelson, HE, 149, *152*
Nelson, HS, 64, *71*
Newhouse, MT, 66, *71*
Newman, GB, 127, *136*
Newman, T, 73, *82*
Newnham, DM, 123, 127, *132*
Nicklas, R, 103, *113*
Nielsen, K, 107, *116*
Niewoehner, DE, 120, 121, 124, *130*, *131*
Nisar, M, 121, 122, *130*, *131*
Nishikawa, M, 19, *28*
Nishimura, K, 62, 63, *70*, *71*, 123, 126, 128, 129, *132*, *133*, *134*
Noah, TL, 172, *183*
Norvald, G, 10, *25*
Nossen, GD, 127, 129, *133*
Novack, AH, 105, *115*
Numa, S, 14, *25*
Nunn, AJ, 106, *115*

O

O'Brien, T, 127, *136*
O'Connor, B, 41, *54*, 137, 141, *150*
O'Connor, BJ, 42, *54*, 63, *70*, 142, 143, 144, *150*

O'Donnell, DE, 124, *132*, 149, *152*
O'Driscoll, BR, 75, 77, 81, *83*
Oda, T, 173, *184*
Oehling, AG, 104, *113*
Ogra, PL, 180, *186*
Okanlami, O, 15, *27*
Okayama, M, 7, 8, 13, 14, 16, 17, *24*, 37, 39, *52*, *53*, 174, *184*
Olen, L, 106, *115*
Ollerenshaw, S, 7, *23*
Olry, R, 4, *23*
Olsen, L, 107, *116*
Olymulder, CG, 21, *29*
Openshaw, PJ, 180, *186*
Ophir, D, 104, *114*
Orgel, A, 94, *98*, 148, *151*
Orgel, HA, 95, *99*
Orson, J, 106, *115*
Osberg, B, 107, *116*
Osler, W, 163, *168*
Ouelette, JJ, 171, *182*

P

Page, CP, 15, 19, *27*, *28*
Palmer, JB, 15, *27*, 33, *50*
Palmer, JD, 34, *51*
Palmer, KNV, 127, *136*
Panthong, A, 160, *168*
Panuska, JR, 48, *55*
Paoletti, P, 148, *151*
Pappas, G, 102, *111*
Pare, PD, 75, 77, 81, *83*
Park, J, 160, *168*
Parker, RA, 127, *136*
Parrino, TA, 106, *115*
Partanen, N, 7, *23*
Pasteline, G, 121, *131*
Patel, H, 42, *54*, 137, 140, *150*
Patel, HJ, 15, *26*, 36, 40, 41, *52*
Patel, K, 171, 173, *182*
Patrick, DM, 68, *72*, 127, 129, *134*
Pattemore, P, 81, *84*
Pattemore, PK, 171, 172, *182*

Pattermore, PK, 103, 109, *112*, *117*
Patterson, NAM, 66, *71*, 126, 127, *135*
Pauwels, R, 121, *131*
Pavia, D, 69, *72*
Pearson, MG, 121, 122, *130*, *131*
Pearson, SB, 42, *54*
Pecho, E, 105, *114*
Pedder, EK, 10, *25*
Pendergast, M, 176, *185*
Pernow, B, 6, *23*
Persson, CGA, 120, *130*
Peset, R, 127, 129, *133*
Pesin, J, 63, 68, 70, 123, 126, *132*, *135*
Peterson, C, 105, *114*
Peterson, GL, 176, *185*
Petrie, GR, 127, *136*
Petty, TL, 62, *70*, 122, *131*
Pfahl, M, 46, *55*
Philip, G, 93, *98*
Phillips, CA, 171, *182*
Phillips, CD, 108, *116*
Piacentini, GL, 81, *85*
Pidoux, H, 159, 163, *168*
Piedimonte, G, 172, *183*
Pierce, RJ, 74, *83*
Pierson, RN, 65, *71*
Pircher, H, 180, *186*
Plaitakis, A, 157, *168*
Pohl, G, 149, *152*
Polak, JM, 4, *23*
Poppius, H, 127, *136*
Posner, M, 107, *116*, 148, *151*
Postma, DS, 127, 129, *133*, 148, *151*
Poukkula, A, 126, *135*
Pouthier-Simon, F, 171, *182*
Pretolani, M, 178, *186*
Pride, NB, 67, *71*, 148, *151*
Prignot, J, 124, 126, *133*
Prince, GA, 172, *183*
Principe, PJ, 33, *50*

Proud, D, 103, 104, *112*, *113*, 172, *183*
Pugsley, JA, 121, *131*

Q

Quereshi, F, 81, *85*

R

Rabe, KF, 19, *28*, 35, *51*, 121, *131*
Racke, K, 15, *26*
Raeburn, D, 19, *28*
Rahman, M, 102, 108, *112*
Rajakulasingam, K, 88, 90, *97*
Rajan, KG, 74, *83*
Rakatosihanaka, J, 18, *28*
Ramers, H, 33, *50*
Ramis, L, 123, 127, 128, *132*
Rammeloo, RHU, 128, *133*
Ramnarine, SI, 39, *53*
Rano, S, 33, *50*
Rao, G, 176, 179, *185*
Raphael, G, 93, *98*
Raphael, GD, 90, 92, 93, *97*
Raphael, GR, 7, 17, 18, *23*
Ratner, P, 148, *151*
Rebuck, AS, 64, 66, 68, 69, *71*, *72*, 75, 77, 81, *83*, 127, 129, *134*, 149, *152*, 165, 166, *169*
Record, FM, 180, *186*
Reddy, H, 3, 8, 11, 15, 16, 18, *22*
Reed, CE, 171, *182*
Reed, G, 127, *136*
Reed, W, 172, *183*
Rees, J, 148, *151*
Rees, PJ, 126, *134*
Rehder, K, 14, *25*
Reichal, R, 41, 42, 43, *54*
Reid, JL, 165, *169*
Reid, LM, 7, *23*
Reinheimer, T, 32, 34, *50*
Reisman, J, 81, *85*

Reissmann, H, 124, *132*
Rennard, SI, 68, *72*, 121, 124, *130*
Reynaert, MS, 75, 81, *84*
Reynolds, S, 74, *83*
Rhoden, KJ, 19, *28*
Rhys Jones, E, 166, *169*
Rich, D, 102, *111*
Richardson, JB, 7, 17, *23*, 59, 60, *69*
Riechl, R, 137, 139, 140, 141, *150*
Rigby, PJ, 172, *183*
Riker, DK, 101, *111*
Rink, E, 87, 88, 90, *96*
Rivard, S, 102, 108, *112*
Rivers, JM, 104, *114*
Roberts, FF, 40, *54*
Roberts, JA, 19, *28*
Roberts, JM, 7, *24*, 32, *49*
Robertson, C, 81, *85*
Robertson, DN, 19, *28*
Robinson, DA, 10, *25*
Rodd, A, 4, *22*
Rodger, IW, 19, *28*
Rodrigues de Miranda, JF, 7, 14, 17, 19, *24, 28*, 32, *50*
Rodwell, F, 148, *151*
Rodwell, P, 75, 77, 78, 80, 81, 82, *84*
Roesler, J, 75, 81, *84*
Roffel, AF, 7, 21, *24*, *29*, 31, 35, 38, 39, *49, 51, 52, 53*
Rogers, DF, 15, *27*, 32, 39, *49, 53*
Rohde, JAL, 32, *49*
Rohode, JAL, 16, *27*
Rominger, KL, 41, 42, 43, *54*, 137, 139, 140, 141, *150*
Roopra, A, 42, *54*
Rosenbaum, LC, 176, *185*
Rosenblatt, MB, 163, *168*
Rossen, RD, 103, *112*
Rossing, TH, 77, 81, *84, 85*
Roszko, P, 148, *151*
Rould, E, 32, 34, *50*
Rousell, J, 19, 20, *28, 29*, 44, 45, 46, 47, 48, 49, *55*

Rousell, JA, 39, 43, *53*
Roux, F, 15, *27*
Roy, A, 104, *113*
Rubenstein, I, 172, *183*
Rubin, A, 126, 129, *133*
Rubino, JR, 102, 108, *112*
Rudnitsky, GS, 73, *82*
Ruffie, C, 178, *186*
Ruffin, RE, 64, *71*, 129, *134*
Russell, MA, 103, *113*
Rystedt, G, 108, *116*

S

Sackner, M, 104, *114*
Sackner, MA, 149, *152*
Said, SI, 4, 7, *22, 23*
Sakethoo, K, 104, *114*
Salmeron, S, 74, *83*
Salorinne, Y, 127, *136*
Salter, HH, 162, 166, 167, *168*
Saltiel, AR, 46, *55*
Salvatori, VA, 93, *98*
Samo, TC, 109, *117*
Sampson, AS, 15, *27*, 33, *50*
Samuel, CE, 180, *186*
Sanderson, G, 81, *84*, 103, *112*, 171, 172, *182*
Sankey, RJ, 106, *115*
Santig, RE, 21, *29*
Saradeth, T, 105, *114*
Saster, A, 106, *115*
Satoh, M, 14, 16, *25*
Sattar, SA, 102, 108, *112*
Saunders, KB, 127, *136*
Saunders, PA, 44, *55*
Sauter, D, 73, *82*
Scarpace, PJ, 172, *183*
Schachter, EN, 137, *150*
Schapowal, A, 104, *113*
Schatz, M, 88, *97*
Schector, EN, 75, *84*
Scheibner, T, 7, *23*

Scheid, A, 176, *185*
Scherrer, M, 165, *169*
Schlick, W, 33, *50*
Schmitz, M, 104, *113*
Schoene, RB, 81, *85*
Schoffstall, JM, 73, *82*
Schofield, BH, 15, *26*, 39, *52*, 178, *186*
Schroeider, R, 15, 20, *26*
Schuh, H, 66, *71*
Schuh, S, 79, 81, *84*, 148, *151*
Schultes, RE, 158, 161, *168*
Schultheis, A, 15, *27*
Schwartz, LB, 180, *187*
Seaver, NA, 32, 34, *50*
Sederberg-Olsen, AE, 108, *116*
Sederberg-Olsen, JF, 108, *116*
Seigel, D, 74, *83*
Sekizawa, K, 172, *183*
Selner, J, 81, *85*
Selner, JC, 88, *96*
Serby, CW, 68, *72*, 121, 124, *130*, 147, *151*
Serra, G, 127, 128, *133*
Sertl, K, 33, *50*
Shah, PKD, 60, *70*
Shannon, FT, 103, *113*
Sheehan, NF, 69, *72*
Shelhamer, JH, 90, *97*, 120, *130*
Shen, T, 37, *52*, 174, *184*
Sheppard, D, 74, *83*
Sheppard, MN, 7, *23*
Shimerlik, MI, 176, *185*
Shimura, S, 14, 16, *25*
Shin, JW, 129, *133*
Shirleaf, J, 73, *82*
Showell, HJ, 177, *185*
Shrestha, M, 127, *136*
Shult, P, 172, *183*
Siafakas, NM, 148, *151*
Siafakis, NM, 67, *71*
Sibald, B, 87, 88, 90, *96*
Siebenlist, U, 46, *55*

Siefken, H, 15, 17, 20, *26*, *27*
Sigurbergsson, F, 180, *186*
Sigurs, N, 180, *186*
Sills, JA, 106, *115*
Silva, G, 149, *152*
Silvers, GW, 122, *131*
Silvers, W, 93, *98*
Simmons, M, 129, *134*
Simon, G, 101, *111*
Simon, JU, 104, *113*
Simons, FER, 74, 75, *83*
Singer, SH, 177, *185*
Sips, AP, 128, *133*
Sjogren, I, 91, *97*
Skomer, DP, 104, *113*
Skorodin, MS, 60, 61, 63, 64, 66, 67, 70, 122, 126, *131*, *132*, 145, 148, *150*
Sledsens, TJ, 63, *70*
Sledsens, TJH, 146, 147, 149, *151*
Sledsens, TJM, 42, *54*
Sliwinski, P, 124, *133*
Slutsky, AS, 18, *28*
Smeets, JJ, 42, *54*, 63, *70*, 145, 146, 147, 149, *151*
Smith, AP, 103, *113*
Smith, D, 129, *134*
Smith, DH, 87, 88, 90, *96*
Smith, DL, 69, *72*, 149, *152*, 165, *169*
Smith, J, 126, *135*
Smith, MBH, 102, 106, *111*
Smith, P, 149, *152*
Smith, WHR, 75, *83*, 129, *134*
Snider, GL, 122, *132*
Solley, GO, 180, *187*
Songsiridej, V, 173, *184*
Sorkness, R, 176, 181, *185*, *187*
Sorrentino, JV, 101, 109, *111*, *117*
Souhrada, JF, 149, *152*
Speck, G, 41, 42, 43, *54*, 137, 139, 140, 141, *150*
Spector, SL, 95, *98*, 103, *112*, *113*
Speers, DM, 171, 173, *182*

Sperber, SJ, 101, 105, 106, 109, *111*, *114*, *115*, *117*
Spitzer, SA, 129, *134*
Spitzer, WO, 78, *84*
Spivey, WH, 73, *82*
Springall, DR, 4, *23*
Springer, TA, 109, *117*
Springthorpe, VS, 102, 108, *112*
Stainforth, JN, 126, *135*
Stark, RM, 68, *72*, 127, 129, *134*
Starke, ID, 127, *136*
Stauton, DE, 109, *117*
Stechschulte, DJ, 15, *27*
Steele, D, 129, *134*
Steinjans, V, 33, *50*
Stenhouse, AC, 171, *182*
Stephens, NL, 120, *130*
Sterk, PJ, 15, *27*
Stewart, JH, 121, *131*
Stjarne, P, 7, 18, *24*, *28*
Stolley, P, 106, *115*
Stone, AA, 103, *113*
Stone, P, 63, *71*
Storms, W, 88, *96*
Stott, EJ, 171, *182*
Stouch, WH, 171, *182*
Stradling, JR, 75, *83*
Strauss, L, 79, *84*
Stubinsky, Y, 177, *185*
Subauste, MC, 172, *183*
Sudlow, MF, 122, *131*
Sugiura, N, 63, *71*, 129, *133*
Suissa, S, 78, *84*
Sulkes, J, 129, *134*
Sullivan, C, 7, *23*
Summers, E, 149, *152*
Summers, Q, 75, 77, *83*
Sundler, F, 7, *23*
Sung, T, 35, 39, *51*
Sung, TC, 11, *25*
Suratt, PM, 63, *70*
Suzuki, F, 173, *184*
Svedmyr, N, 77, *84*

Swensen, CA, 171, *182*
Sybrecht, GW, 33, *50*

T

Tacke, R, 8, *24*
Tadjkarimi, S, 15, *26*, 36, 40, 41, *52*, 137, 140, *150*
Takahashi, T, 36, 40, 41, 42, *52*, *54*
Takahaski, T, 137, 140, *150*
Takehashi, T, 15, *26*
Tamaoki, J, 172, 177, *183*
Tandon, MK, 121, *131*
Tang, OT, 127, *136*
Tang, W, 104, *113*
Tarala, RA, 75, 77, *83*
Tarara, JE, 15, *27*
Tashkin, D, 147, *151*
Tashkin, DP, 66, *71*, 121, 127, 129, *130*, *134*, *136*
Tavakol, M, 73, *82*
Tavakoli, S, 120, *130*
Taylor, DR, 121, *131*
Taylor, J, 147, *151*
Taylor, JA, 105, *115*
Taylor, RJ, 75, 77, 81, *83*
Taylor, WC, 160, *168*
Teichgradeber, J, 93, *98*
Teisman, AC, 38, *52*
Temple, WP, 123, 126, *132*
Templeton, DJ, 48, *55*
Ten Berge, RE, 21, *29*, 38, *52*
Thomas, P, 121, *131*
Thompson, HS, 156, 158, *167*
Thomson, NC, 19, *28*
Timmers, MC, 15, *27*
Tinkelman, DG, 106, *115*, 148, *151*
Togias, A, 93, *98*
Toivanen, M, 7, *23*
Tokuyama, K, 15, *27*, 32, *49*
Tom-Moy, M, 33, *50*
Toogood, JH, 66, *71*, 126, 127, *135*
Town, GI, 75, 77, 78, 80, 81, 82, *84*

Town, L, 148, *151*
Towse, LJ, 42, *54*, 63, *70*, 142, 143, 144, *150*
Tramontana, JA, 156, *167*
Traunecker, W, 137, 139, 140, 141, *150*
Travnecker, W, 41, 42, 43, *54*
Trechsel, K, 165, *169*
Trouseau, A, 159, 163, *168*
Trumpp-Kallmeyer, S, 10, *25*
Tsukino, M, 129, *134*
Turner-Warwick, M, 127, *136*
Tuxe, K, 6, *23*
Tyrell, RJ, 102, *111*
Tyrrell, D, 104, *114*
Tyrrell, DA, 103, *113*
Tyrrell, DAJ, 109, *117*

U

Uddman, R, 7, *23*
Ukena, D, 33, *50*
Ullah, M, 127, *136*
Umeno, E, 172, *183*
Utell, MJ, 104, *113*, 171, 173, *183*

V

Valentine, MD, 148, *151*
Valletta, EA, 81, *85*
Van Amsterdam, RGM, 35, *51*
Van de Mark, T, 127, 129, *133*
Van der Meer, FJ, 15, *27*
Van der Straeten, M, 121, *131*
Van der Veen, H, 15, *27*
Van Ginneken, CAM, 7, 14, *24*, 32, *50*
Van Koppen, CJ, 7, 14, 19, *24*, *28*, 32, *50*
Van Megen, YJB, 17, *28*
Vargaftig, BB, 178, *186*
Vaughan, TR, 64, *71*
Veki, I, 90, *97*
Vermeire, P, 148, *151*

Vermiere, P, 67, *71*
Viljanen, AA, 127, *136*
Voelker, H, 77, *84*
Vogel, Z, 10, *25*
Von Barbeleben, RS, 17, *27*
Vrtis, RF, 171, *182*

W

Wagenmann, M, 91, *98*
Wald, FD, 63, *70*
Wald, FDM, 42, *54*, 128, *133*, 145, 146, 147, 149, *151*
Walker, FB, 63, *70*
Wallen, O, 165, *169*
Walsh, JJ, 179, *186*
Walshaw, M, 121, *130*
Walters, J, 73, *82*
Walti, S, 180, *186*
Wang, CD, 10, *25*
Wang, J, 120, *130*
Wang, Y, 48, *55*
Wanner, A, 121, *131*
Waon-Toi, H, 81, *85*
Ward, JK, 42, *54*, 137, 140, *150*
Ward, MJ, 66, *71*, 74, 75, 77, *83*, *84*, 129, *134*, 148, *151*
Warner, JO, 66, *71*
Warshauer, D, 172, *183*
Waters, ATM, 163, *168*
Watson, N, 3, 8, 10, 11, 15, 16, 18, 19, *22*, *24*, *28*, 35, 36, 39, *51*
Watson, WTA, 74, 75, *83*
Webb, BL, 20, *29*
Webb, BLJ, 44, 45, *55*
Webb, DR, 88, *97*
Webb, KA, 124, *132*, 149, *152*
Weber, RW, 64, *71*
Wecker, M, 93, *98*
Wecker, MT, 108, *116*, 148, *151*
Wegner, RE, 121, 129, *131*
Wehinger, C, 33, *50*
Weigand, GW, 173, *184*
Weipple, G, 107, *115*

Welliver, RC, 171, 180, *182*, *186*
Wellman, JJ, 63, *70*
Wentges, BTR, 17, *28*
Wentworth, CE, 76, 77, 81, *84*
Wess, J, 8, 10, *24*, *25*
Wesseling, G, 127, *136*
Wessler, I, 15, *26*
West, S, 106, *115*
Whicker, SD, 19, *28*
White, M, 91, *98*
White, MV, 91, *98*
Widdicombe, JG, 60, *69*
Williams, CL, 15, *27*
Williams, SJ, 74, *83*
Wills-Karp, M, 15, *26*, 38, *52*, 148, *152*, 174, 178, *184*
Wilson, MH, 106, *115*
Wilson, NM, 42, *54*
Winner, SJ, 74, *83*
Winter, B, 107, *116*
Winter, JH, 123, 127, *132*
Winther, B, 103, 107, *112*, *116*
Wirz, P, 105, *114*
Witek, TJ, 137, 147, *150*, *151*
Wolf, D, 15, 20, *26*
Wolfe, JD, 129, *134*
Wolkove, N, 75, 77, 81, *83*
Wood, C, 102, *111*, 148, *151*
Wood, CC, 93, *98*
Wood, IC, 43, *54*
Wood, PB, 108, *116*, 148, *151*
Woolcock, A, 7, *23*
Wouters, EFM, 127, *136*
Wrana, JL, 46, *55*
Wright, E, 121, 124, *130*
Wright, RH, 18, *28*, 91, *97*

X

Xiao, HQ, 36, *51*, 178, 179, *185*, *186*

Y

Yacoub, MH, 15, *26*, 36, 40, 41, *52*
Yamamura, HI, 14, 16, 17, *25*, 32, 33, 34, *50*, *51*
Yan, S, 124, *133*
Yang, B, 17, *28*
Yang, CM, 11, 20, *25*, *29*, 35, 39, *51*
Yarkony, KA, 177, 179, *185*
Yarosh, CA, 34, *51*
Ye, DYC, 17, *27*
Yen-Lieberman, BR, 104, *114*
Yernault, JC, 148, *151*
Yocub, MH, 137, 140, *150*
Yoshitomi, T, 36, *52*, 174, *184*
Yost, BL, 39, *53*, 174, 178, *184*
Yost, BY, 15, *26*
Yu, SM, 102, *111*

Z

Zaagsma, J, 7, 21, *24*, *29*, 31, 35, 38, 39, *49*, *51*, *52*, *53*
Zarembo, JE, 105, *114*
Zaritsky, A, 81, *85*
Zegarelli, E, 148, *151*
Zeiger, RS, 88, *97*
Zheng, T, 173, *183*
Zhu, Z, 104, *113*
Zimmerman, PV, 126, *134*, *135*
Zinny, M, 126, *135*
Zinny, MA, 148, *151*

SUBJECT INDEX

A

Acetylcholine (ACh), 3, 4, 175
Adhesion molecule (VLA-4), 39
Adjunctive role in status asthmaticus, 66
Adrenergic agents, 64, 65
Allergen challenge, 38
Allergen inhalation, 65
Allergic rhinitis, 88
Analgesic/anti-inflammatory agents, 105
Antibiotics, 108
Anticholinergic agents, 61
Anticholinergic agents as bronchodilators
  long-term effects of, 68
  side effects of, 69
Anticholinergic/beta-agonist bronchodilator combination, 128
Anticholinergic/beta agonist combination therapy, 129
Anticholinergic bronchodilators (smoke), 160
Anticholinergics in combination in COPD, 119
Anticholinergics in COPD, 121
Anticholinergic therapy, subgroups who derive particular benefit, 80
Antihistamine/decongestant combinations, 106
Antihistamines, 106
Anti-inflammatory agents, 108
Antimuscarinics, historical aspects of, 155
Antitussives, 105
Asthma, 65
  most-severe, 81
Asthma cigarettes, 165
Atropine, 40, 62
Atropine methonitrate, 63

B

β-adrenergic blockers, 37
Bronchodilation, 143
  onset and duration of, 64

C

Carbachol (1 mM), 44, 65
Ceramide, 48

Cholinergic ganglia, 4
Cholinergic mechanisms in perennial rhinitis, 91
Cholinergic muscarinic receptors, 60
Cholinergic tone, 122
Chronic obstructive pulmonary disease (COPD), 66, 67, 119, 120, 121, 145
  mechanisms of, 120
Cold dry air, 65
Combined bronchodilator therapy, 122
Combivent, 62
Common cold, 101, 104
  contributing or exacerbating factors, 103
  management of, 104
  pharmacologic remedies, 105
Cyclohexamide, 49
Cytokines, 46, 47

D

Darifenacin (UK-88,525), 17, 41
Datura, 156
Datura poisoning, 157
Datura stramonium, 156
Decongestants, 106
Downregulation, 13
Duration of action, 64

E

Efferent nerves, 4
Eosinophil major basic protein (MBP), 6, 39, 179

F

Fixed combinations, 128

G

Ganglionic autoreceptors, 15
Glycopyrrolate bromide (Robinul), 63

Glycosylation of the M_2 receptor, 176
G-protein-binding region, 12
G-protein-related receptors, 10
Growth factors, 46

H

Histamine, 65
Historical aspects of antimuscarinics, 155
Human pharmacology and early clinical trials, 142
Hyperresponsiveness, 18

I

Improvements in clinical outcomes, 78
Incubation period, 103
Inflammatory responses to viral infections, 177
Influenza virus, 38
Inhaled ipratropium bromide
  effect on maximally employed beta-agonist therapy, 77
  use in acute asthma, 80
Inhibitor G-proteins, 13
Inhibitory M_2 autoreceptors, 15
Interactions between atopy and viral infections, 178
Interleukin-1β (IL-1β), 47
Intranasal ipratropium bromide, 94
Investigational therapy, 109
Iodopindolol, 44
Ipratropium bromide, 40, 41, 62, 63, 74, 107
  augmenting the effect of beta-agonist therapy, 75
  optimal dose in acute severe asthma, 75
  0.5 mg of ipratropium in association with 2.5 vs. 5 mg salbutamol, 82

Subject Index

K

Kinins, 104

L

Long-term effects of anticholinergic agents, 68

M

Methacholine, 65, 92
Methacholine challenge, 43, 144
Most-severe asthma, 81
Muscarinic antagonists, 18
Muscarinic autoreceptors, 36
Muscarinic receptors, 8, 9, 19, 21, 31, 91
   M_1 receptors, 7, 8, 9, 12, 13, 32, 33, 61, 91
      4-DAMP, 8, 9, 42
      L-689.660, 9
      McN-A343, 9, 32
      pirenzepine, 8, 9, 14, 32, 33, 34
      pilocarpine, 9, 15, 37
      telenzepine, 9, 32, 34
   M_2 receptors, 7, 8, 9, 13, 14, 16, 19, 21, 32, 35, 43, 44, 61, 174, 176, 181
      AFDX-116, 8, 9, 32
      betanechol, 9
      receptor dysfunction, 38, 176, 177
      gallamine, 8, 9, 15, 32, 36
      gene expression, 178
      himbascine, 9, 10
      methoctramine, 9, 15, 32, 41, 42
      pilocarpine, 9, 15, 32, 37
   M_3 receptors, 7, 8, 9, 12, 14, 16, 21, 32, 39, 61, 91, 173
      4-DAMP, 8, 9, 32, 39, 42
      hexahydrosiladifenidol (HHSIF), 9, 32, 39
      L-689.660, 9
      zamifenacin, 9

[Muscarinic receptors]
   M_4 receptors, 8, 9, 13, 17, 40, 43
      himbascine, 9, 10
      McN-A343, 9
      methoctramine, 9, 42
   M_5 receptors, 9, 12, 17, 40
Muscarinic receptor structure, 10
Muscarinic receptor subtypes, 91, 173

N

Nasal cholinergic reflexes, 17
Neuraminidase, 6
Neurokinin type 3 subtype receptors, 5
Neurologic factors, 104
Neuropeptide Y (NPY), 5
Nicotinic cholinergic receptors, 34
Nicotinic receptors, 4
Nightshade family (Solanaceae), 155
Nitric oxide synthase (NOS), 4
Nociceptive C-fibers, 91
Nociceptive neuron, 6
Nonadrenergic, noncholinergic (NANC) system, 60
Nonpharmacologic remedies, 104

O

Oxitropium bromide (Oxivent), 40, 43, 63
Oxivent, 63
O_3, 6

P

Parasympathetic innervation, 4, 5
Pathophysiology of perennial rhinitis, 89
Pediatric asthma, 66
Perennial nonallergic rhinitis, 89
Perennial rhinitis, 87, 94
Pharmacology, 138
PHM, 2, 6
Placebo effect, 95

Postrecovery changes in M_2 receptor function, 181
Prostaglandin dependency, 16
Protection against broncospastic stimuli, 65
Protein kinase C, 45
Psychogenic bronchospasm, 65
Psychotropic uses of antimuscarinic botanicals, 157

Q

Quaternary ammonium agents, 69
Quaternary ammonium muscarinic receptor antagonists, 93

R

Revatropate (UK-112,116), 17
Reversibility to beta agonists in patients with COPD, 120
Rhinitis, late-phase reaction of, 90
Rhodopsin family, 10
Robinul, 63

S

Side effects of anticholinergic agents, 69
Solanaceae, 155
Stramonium, 165
Sympathetic nervous system, 4
Systemic antihistamines, combination with, 95
Systemic symptoms, 103

T

Tachykinins, 6, 177
  role of in virus-induced M_2 receptor dysfunction, 177

Tertiary ammonium agents, 69
Theophylline in COPD, 121, 129
Tiotropium bromide (Ba 679), 41, 42, 43, 63, 137, 144
  effect on methacholine challenge, 144
  effect in patients with COPD, 145
  multiple-dose, dose-ranging study, 146
  potential role in clinical practice, 147
  single-dose, dose-ranging study, 146
T_m helices, 10
Tolerance, 64
Transforming growth factor-((TGF-β), 46
Tumor necrosis factor α (TNF-α), 47

U

Upper respiratory infections, 101
  pathogenesis and epidemiology, 102
  prevention, 109
Use of inhaled ipratropium bromide in acute asthma, 80

V

Vasoactive intestinal peptide (VIP), 4, 6, 7
Viral infections, 81, 171, 176, 177, 178
Virus-induced changes in airway function, 172
Virus-induced parasympathetic hyperresponsiveness, 173

Z

Zinc lozenges, 105

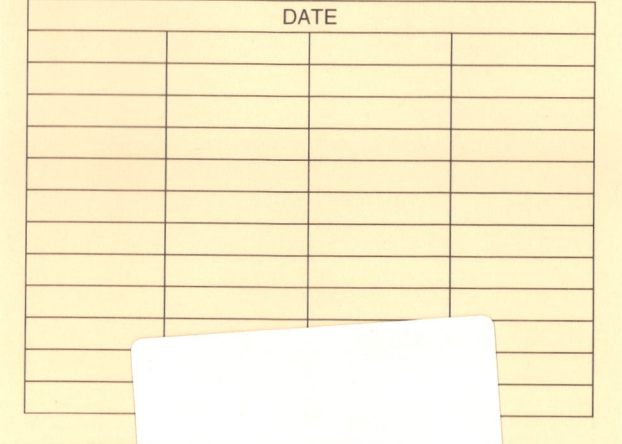